THE SIMPLE FACTS

FACT: On average, people sixty-five and over are given fourteen prescriptions a year and use two or three a day.

FACT: During hospital stays, older people are given an average of ten different drugs.

FACT: The more drugs you use, the more likely you are to have adverse reactions.

FACT: Nearly twenty-five percent of hospital admissions for older people are due to adverse reactions to drugs. Most of these situations are avoidable.

FACT: THE SAFE MEDICINE BOOK can help you manage your medication, take control of your health, and make the most of the best years of your life.

THE SAFE
MEDICINE
BOOK

Kathryn Watterson

Foreword by Robert N. Butler, M.D.

Published with the cooperation and consultation of the Gerald and May Ellen Ritter Department of Geriatrics and Adult Development, Mount Sinai School of Medicine, Mount Sinai Hospital.

IVY BOOKS • NEW YORK

Ivy Books
Published by Ballantine Books

Library of Congress Catalog Card Number: 86-48011

ISBN 0-8041-0861-7

Manufactured in the United States of America

First Trade Edition: April 1988
First Mass Market Edition: March 1992

*This book is dedicated to
my father, Robert P. Watterson, M.D.,
a maverick and a pioneering geriatrician,
who would have enjoyed seeing so many of his visions
realized.*

Contents

Foreword

Kathryn Watterson's *Safe Medicine Book* is required reading for people who want to become better informed consumers of prescription and nonprescription drugs, and it is decidedly in their interest to do so as they get older.

As Ms. Watterson so rightly points out, people who do not take the time to learn about the medications they are taking can end up misusing the very things that could save and enhance the quality of their lives. It's not unusual, for example, for older persons to share medications with friends whose symptoms seem similar, but whose conditions and treatment may be quite different. Patients sometimes decide to stop taking their prescribed medication after they begin to feel better. However, feeling better doesn't automatically mean that the condition being treated has been eradicated. Others have so many bottles of pills in the house that they get them confused and end up picking up the wrong one, or they take pills that have been sitting in the medicine cabinet way past their expiration date, when their effectiveness has decreased and their potential for hurting the patient has increased.

Educated consumers are more likely to avoid such drug errors, to distinguish between normal and adverse effects of the drugs they are taking, and to report unusual or unpleasant drug reactions to their physicians. That's precisely why it's so important to study *The Safe*

Medicine Book. Kathryn Watterson's extensive research has made it an indispensable source of information for people who recognize the need to get involved in their own and their family's health care. It should be kept within easy reach and consulted whenever necessary.

As we age, it becomes increasingly important to learn about the medications we take. Side effects may be different in older people because of changes in metabolism and excretion. Moreover, there is a tendency for fat to replace muscle, which causes the effects of fat-soluble medications to last longer. Doctors often need to prescribe several drugs for their older patients, and "polypharmacy" can lead to adverse drug interactions, hospitalization, and, in the most serious cases, death.

Only recently, since 1983 to be exact, has the Food and Drug Administration taken serious steps toward establishing guidelines for studying the effects of drugs in older people, and these guidelines are now on the verge of becoming official. Traditionally, drug testing, including measuring the level of drugs in the blood, observing liver and kidney functions, and post-marketing followup—called Phase IV marketing—was reserved for the younger population, with age sixty-five as the cutoff point. No more. Now there is interest in older persons, due in part to the fact that the proportion of people over sixty-five in our population, which has been rising steadily since the first few decades of this century, will continue to increase well into the twenty-first century, when over 20 percent of the total U.S. population will be sixty-five or older. This increased attention is also due to the fact that more and more people are living longer, healthier, more productive lives, and, in many cases, their longevity has been helped by better, more effective drugs—in fact, in the U.S., people over sixty-five consume some 25 percent of prescription medications.

While there's reason to rejoice at the attention older consumers are now getting, the fact is that physicians, pharmacologists, pharmaceutical companies, pharmacists, clinical pharmacists, and the Food and Drug Administration are still a long way from knowing all we need to know about drugs in older people. That's why it's essential for patients—and their families—to take an active role in their health care and not rely entirely on the imperfect knowledge of "experts."

Robert N. Butler, M.D.
New York, N.Y.

A Note to the Reader

I've written this book as a commonsense introduction to the concepts involved in aging and using medications. Whether you are sixty-five or older, or whether you are the child or grandchild of someone that age, I hope this book will give you new insights and persuade you to pause and think about what you're doing before you take any medicine.

When I began my research, I knew very little about chemistry, about drugs, or about aging. I was not a medical writer—and that's the way my editors wanted it. They insisted that if I could make sense out of this subject, other people would understand it, too. *The Safe Medicine Book* is the result of my efforts to come to terms with information that was complex, confusing, and sometimes absolutely contradictory. When it comes to aging and medicine, many "facts" are relative, if not controversial, among medical professionals. Even "safe medicine" is a relative term. No medicine is safe unless it is prescribed and taken appropriately, and even then, drugs can sometimes act quite unpredictably and harmfully within a particular individual. What is normal for one older person may not be normal for the next.

It became clear to me as I worked on this book that many people—patients and physicians alike—simply do not make a distinction between being sick and being old. All too often I heard stories about situations in

which people had severe reactions to medications that
were misinterpreted by doctors, friends, and families
as "signs of aging." Sometimes these reactions to medications were physical and sometimes psychological—
but symptoms that ranged from stumbling to extreme
confusion were instantly "cured" when the older person was taken off the offending medication.

I started my interviews for this book in rural Kansas,
which has a larger percentage of people sixty-five and
over than any other nonmetropolitan area in the United
States. I continued my research in New York, New Jersey, and Pennsylvania, where I talked with many older
people and their physicians, pharmacists, nurses, and
social workers. I also interviewed people throughout
the country by telephone. The quality of life of the people I interviewed ranged from poor to excellent, as did
their energy, income, productivity, and health.

The many people I interviewed will be delighted if
the stories and information they shared make you more
aware, more assertive, more questioning, and more
careful when it comes to managing your medications. I
hope this book will serve as a catalyst for making you
a more informed consumer, and that it will give you an
approach and an attitude toward your health that will
serve you well.

                                        Kathryn Watterson
                                        Princeton, New Jersey

A Note on Usage

When I use the term *older people* or *the elderly*, I'm referring to people sixty-five and older.

I have used either *he* or *she* when referring to physicians, pharmacists, nurses, and other health-care professionals. When I use *he* or *she* exclusively in a general statement, I am referring to health-care professionals of both sexes.

In many cases, I've changed names and places to protect the patients or doctors who asked not to be identified. Where I have changed the names, I've put quotes around the name.

In referring to drugs, I've used generic names (which are not capitalized) and, for the most part, put brand names (which are capitalized) in parentheses. When I have used either the brand name or the generic name, you'll know the difference by whether or not the name of the medication is capitalized. The generic name is the "official" name of the drug and is often descriptive of the drug's chemical composition or class. Every drug has a generic name assigned in the early stages of its development. However, brand names are trade names used exclusively by the drug company that invents and produces the drug.

Acknowledgments

I couldn't have written this book without the advice and direction of medical professionals. For bringing their experience, expertise, intellect, and time to the content of this book, I am especially appreciative of Sylvia McBurnie, assistant professor of Nursing at the State University of New York, The Health Science Center at Brooklyn's College of Nursing; Dr. Barbara Otto; Dr. Diane Meier of Mount Sinai's Geriatric Clinic; and Dr. Michael Freedman, director of the Division of Geriatrics at New York University Medical Center. I also appreciate the time and contributions made by Mia Oberlink, Dr. David Lowenthal, Dr. Caleb Finch, Dr. William Gershell, Dr. Peter Lamy, Dr. Bernard Mehl, Dr. Andrew Lautin, Dr. Teruko Neuwalder, Mr. Randall Wright, Mr. Mel Atlas, Ms. Caroline Robb, Dr. Douglas Young, and many other medical professionals who generously shared their knowledge with me.

Throughout the process of writing this book, Dianne B. Stern's research, anecdotes, and humor were of great assistance to me. Madeline Feinberg, pharmacist and director of the Elder-Health program at the University of Maryland's School of Pharmacy, also added to the depth and substance of this book.

In addition, I want to thank Lynne Payer and Marlene Charnizon for their editorial help, and Julie Govert Walter and the staff of the Area Agency on Aging in Manhattan, Kansas, Pat Van Atta Embers, Marlene

Ascherman, Jacqueline David, Tony Auth, Rorrey Za-
hourek, and Donna Calame—all of whom contributed
to my understanding of the larger picture.

Special thanks goes to my mother, Grace Watterson
Landis, and to my aunts and uncles and the many other
older people who enriched this book by sharing stories
of their own medical experiences with me.

Further acknowledgment goes to my editors, Ann La
Farge and Joëlle Delbourgo, to Jane Bess, who shep-
herded it through its final stages, to Sara Miller, for her
superb copyediting of this edition, and to my agents,
Connie Clausen and Guy Kettelhack.

Gratitude and love to Lee Gruzen, Marie Stoner, and
Alice Watterson, to my husband, Ron Sitts, and my
son, Zachary David, who helped me and gave me balance, fun, and laughter in the process.

CHAPTER 1

★

An Overview—
Aging and the Use of Medicine

"I do not wish two diseases, one nature-made and one man-made."

NAPOLEON

"I don't buy medicines, I *bowl*!" says Alice Green, who owns and operates an art gallery she opened nine years ago at the age of eighty. "I haven't paid a doctor for anything except a physical in years, and I don't ever spend a penny at the drugstore, not even on aspirin. Some of my relatives used to criticize me for spending money on bowling. I always told them I'd rather spend my money on bowling than on the doctor. Now that they've been going to the hospital for all kinds of tests, and paying for all kinds of medicines, they're beginning to get the idea."

Like her mother, who died at the age of 104, Alice Green is an excellent example of what it means to age naturally and comfortably, free from disease. Trim and fit at five foot three inches, Alice bowls at the local bowling alley in McPherson, Kansas, four times a week—two of those times with a league bowling team that wears yellow shirts emblazoned with "Alice's Gallery" on the back.

"Most of what they tell you about being old is bunk," Alice says, her luminous green eyes flashing with humor as she stretches up to hang a painting on the wall. "Don't believe what anybody tells you when they say they can't remember or can't do something 'cause they're old.' It might be because they're sick, but it

1

doesn't have a darn thing to do with being old. Old is all in your mind and the way you look at it. People shouldn't use their age as an excuse for things. It gives getting old a bad name!''

Although many eighty-nine-year-olds are not as vigorous and disease-free as Alice Green, she is more typical of people over sixty-five than stereotypes would lead us to believe. "Really?" you might ask, disbelieving. "Old people aren't that healthy!" Wrong. Although some older people do fit the stereotype of the frail, shrunken person being wheeled through the nursing home, with life's memories captured in small framed pictures on faded hand-crocheted doilies beside the bed, in fact, only a small percentage of older people face that sort of fate.

The truth is that less than 5 percent of all the people in this country who are sixty-five and over live in nursing homes. *The other 95 percent live in the community,* and more than 81 percent of them are fully ambulatory and independent. (By the way, the 14 percent who are not fully mobile are largely cared for by their own spouses or children—making the myth that families abandon their old people patently untrue.)

If you're sixty-five or older, the prospects for your continued good health, normal activity, and long life are vastly better than they're commonly portrayed. While a large number of people in your age group do have at least one and sometimes two or three persistent physical problems, many of these chronic ailments are not particularly troublesome. Having high blood pressure is potentially very debilitating, for instance, but if it's well managed, it won't be as troublesome to you on a day-to-day basis at age seventy as bursitis is to a forty-year-old.

"I've had hypertension for years," says seventy-seven-year-old "Amy Chan" of Phoenix, Arizona, "and I feel it's very well controlled. When I started taking medication for it, my doctor gave me various samples and I didn't always respond well to them. I don't think he handled that very well. But now, for the past fifteen years, I've taken two Diazide a day. I never worry about my blood pressure shooting up. I have a lot of confidence that I'll never have a stroke. It's nothing to worry about, but it's something to keep under control and give attention to.

"It used to be that there wasn't any medication for hypertension. Six out of nine of my siblings also have hypertension and it's not in the least bothersome to them. But our mother died of a stroke, and our older brother, Tom, died in his forties before hypertensive medication was available. He was a doctor—and he ended up with kidney damage that killed him. Our oldest brother, Will, had a sympathectomy—that was the surgery they did to prolong the life of a person who had hypertension. He lived ten years after the surgery and then got on medication that gave him another ten years. The rest of us have been more fortunate because now blood pressure can be so well controlled by diet and medicine. . . ."

As Amy's perspective demonstrates, there's been a lot of change from the way things used to be. If we'd lived at the turn of the century, most of us would have thought ourselves lucky if we lived past infancy to the age of sixty-five, let alone rolled our eyes, rotated our ankles, danced or played handball at the age of eighty-two. In 1900, only one-fourth of the population survived their sixty-fifth year, whereas in 1980, almost 70 percent did so. Eight out of ten of today's babies can expect to live well into their seventies and eighties, and the American Association for the Advancement of Science predicts that babies in the next century can expect to live an average of ninety-five years.

Additionally, the quality of life itself has changed for older people. Today the definition of "old" is not what it used to be. Rather than being a simple matter of chronology, "old age" today is defined by one's degree of health and hardiness. This means that for many of us, old age doesn't start until we're well into our seventies, eighties, or even our nineties. If you look around, you'll see many white-haired people jogging around the track in their running sneakers, pushing baskets down the aisles of supermarkets, swinging their tennis racquets, and pedaling their bikes. If it seems you're noticing more people with white or gray hair than you ever saw before, you're right. Today, more than thirty-one million people—12.5 percent of our nation's population—are over sixty-five.

According to the United Nations, the number of older people in the world will double by the year 2030, when one out of every five people will be sixty-five or over. The Bureau of the Census projects that by the turn of the century there will be more than sixteen million people over the age of eighty-five in the United States alone. At a recent meeting of gerontologists, Congressman Claude Pepper announced that, at the age of eighty-five, he was delighted to be a member of the fastest growing group in our population. "Being part of the over-eighty-five group in this country is like being a pioneer," he said. "It's a privilege to belong to it! Recently, I had lunch with a group of centurians. The youngest was one hundred and the oldest was one hundred and twelve. One doctor I met from New Jersey who goes to his office every day is one hundred and three."

"This is the first century of old age," says Dr. Robert Butler, chairman of the Ritter Department of Geriatrics and Adult Development at Mount Sinai School of Medicine. "What used to be the privilege of the few has become the destiny of many." Dr. Butler, a distinguished physician and gerontologist, was the first director of the National Institute on Aging in 1976. He won a Pulitzer Prize that same year for his book *Why Survive? Being Old in America*. Dr. Butler smiles when he speaks about the prospects of today's baby boomers hitting Golden Pond. "By the time they hit Golden Pond, they will make up 20 percent of the population. They'll be one out of every five people in this country, and they will constitute about 35 percent of the voting public. That's going to be a powerful group! What we're seeing is a longevity revolution of individual survival, and a longevity revolution of populations as a whole."

Basically, we're living better and we're living longer. Most of the increase in life expectancy, according to Dr. James W. Davis, Jr., chief of geriatric services at the University of California at Los Angeles Medical Center, is due to public-health measures. These include making childbirth safer for both babies and mothers, taking better care of children, and immunizing them during childhood, as well as having better sanitation, better nutrition, less dangerous work, and fewer accidents in the work place. Medical research and treatment have also made an impact. In the past twenty years, there's been a 25 percent drop in deaths from heart attacks, and a 40 percent drop in deaths from strokes, due in large part to a revolution in heart drugs that have lowered mortality and morbidity from heart attacks and heart disease, to the recognition and treatment of hypertension, and most likely to changes in diet and exercise, decreased cholesterol, and a reduction in cigarette smoking. Properly used medications—antibiotics in particular—have been visible heroes in prolonging life and adding to its quality. They've been part of a phenomenal pharmaceutical and medical unfolding that's taken place during this century. We now have thousands and thousands of medications to treat chronic conditions and acute illnesses. Many of them work so effectively to cure and to heal that they border on the miraculous. Whereas many people used to die regularly from diphtheria, polio, smallpox, tuberculosis, syphilis, and even measles, now we can be inoculated against, or cured of, those diseases.

It wouldn't be surprising if, within our lifetimes—or at least within the lifetimes of our children—scientists also learned through yet-to-be-discovered preventions or treatments, how to eliminate osteoporosis, arthritis, diabetes, heart diseases, high blood pressure, cancer, AIDS, Parkinson's disease, and even Alzheimer's disease. It may also be that within another twenty to thirty years antiaging drugs will be popped like vitamins to slow down the processes of declining energy, graying hair, and wrinkled skin. Longevity drugs may eventually even increase our potential life spans from the present limit of about 115 years to 140 years or more.

MAGIC GONE AWRY—DRUG CRISIS AMONG THE ELDERLY

That's the good news. In the meantime, however, there's a downside to the benefits we've been reaping from medications. Right now in the United States, older people are experiencing a drug crisis of epidemic proportions. This drug crisis is not a result of shooting heroin or sniffing cocaine. The problems come from the improper prescribing by doctors and the improper use by patients of drugs such as Coumadin, digitalis, methyldopa, Tagamet, Aldomet, reserpine/hydrochlorothiazide, potassium, or even aspirin—often useful drugs that have been prescribed to help, not to harm you.

The problems from misusing medications are an enormous threat to your health and longevity; a threat that's far more serious in the numbers of people it affects than any single illness. The misuse of those same medications that improve the quality of your life can also threaten it. Studies show that older people are more vulnerable to errors in the administration of drugs than any other age group. While there's no evidence that older people make more drug errors than younger people, the bad news is that people with older bodies run a much higher risk of side effects, adverse drug reactions, overdosing, illness, injury, hospitalization, and deaths caused by medications than younger people do. The costs to older people economically, physically, and emotionally when they run into trouble from their medicines are staggering.

If you're over sixty-five, you probably already realize that these problems are common; they happen to hundreds of thousands of people every year. Among people you know, they're everyday stories. It's rare to run into anyone over sixty-five who *doesn't* have a horror story about adverse reactions to a drug or its interaction with another medicine that made them or their spouse or their good friend sick.

Recently, at a professional luncheon, I heard of the following situations:

- A steady, sensible, and very kindhearted eighty-one-year-old woman had been wandering the halls of the hospital, hallucinating and screaming obscenities. This woman, who had always been a happy and emotionally generous person, was calling her niece a slut and a whore, cursing her deceased husband, and, according to her daughter, "talking like you would talk if you were in a horrible, ugly dream." The doctor had her strapped down because she was becoming a danger to others and herself. When her granddaughter asked if this could be happening in response to a medication, the doctor took her off the new heart medicine he had prescribed. Within forty-eight hours, she was normal again.

- An independent, feisty lawyer, age seventy-nine, became so depressed that his wife thought he was suicidal. He would get up in the morning out of habit, but within twenty minutes he would crawl back into bed, curl up in a fetal position, and tell her he was just waiting to die. When his wife called the doctor, she was told to stop giving him Captopril, a medication for hypertension that he had been taking for a month. It turned out that he was overdosed; he needed less than half the amount he had been prescribed. Within four days of being off the medication, he felt chipper once again.

- An eighty-four-year-old woman who had just returned from a tour in China began hemorrhaging while walking to the grocery store. She was rushed to the emergency room and into surgery for bleeding ulcers. She had taken aspirin during her walking tour in China to keep pain out of her knees and hadn't always had liquid to drink with it. On the trip home, and again after arriving, she'd taken more aspirin, which had caused the bleeding.

Clearly, medicines, if not prescribed and used properly, can be as dangerous as the disease itself, and even more so if they cause you to be misdiagnosed, hospitalized, or seriously injured. A known fact about this drug crisis is that the more medicines you take, the more likely you are to get into trouble with them.

If you're over sixty-five, you're in an age group that consumes more prescription medications per person than any other group in the United States. While Alice Green may embody the lively spirit of older people, she's the exception, not the rule, when it comes to her independence from medications. Unlike Alice, approximately two-thirds of those of you over the age of sixty-five in the United States use nonprescription drugs on a regular basis. And although you and other people over the age of sixty-five represent only 12.5 percent of the population, it's estimated that you use from 33.3 percent to 39 percent of the 1.7 billion prescription drugs sold annually in this country. This means older adults use a total of *at least* 567 million prescriptions a year.

Altogether, Americans spent nearly $29 billion as outpatients in 1989 for prescription drugs, according to the Health Care Financing Administration. Extrapolating from that figure, we can estimate that older adults spend from $10 billion to $14 billion annually for prescription drugs on an outpatient basis alone.

It's estimated that by the year 2000, people sixty-five and older will consume *50 percent* of all prescription drugs. A significant reason for this widespread use is that today, diseases, along with appropriate therapy for them, have been more specifically defined, and a much wider range of effective drugs are available. Let's look at the drug picture as it exists today for people sixty-five and older:

- Two-thirds of those who live in the community use a daily average of two to three prescriptions on a regular basis.
- Nearly four out of every ten older people use five or more different prescriptions on a regular basis, while one out of five regularly uses seven or more prescriptions at one time.
- On the average, Medicare beneficiaries are given 16.5 prescriptions a year at the average cost of $18.22 per prescription, according to the Health Care Financing Administration.
- When hospitalized, older people are given an average of ten different drugs during each stay in the hospital.
- Altogether, older people spend an average of $300 per person a year for their prescription medications alone. Considering that most older people live on fixed incomes—one-sixth have incomes below the poverty level—this is a large chunk of their finances.

* * *

If spending billions of dollars on prescription drugs produced good health, it would probably be worth it. But it's not that simple.

BIG INVESTMENT, DUBIOUS RETURNS

No one knows for sure the full dimensions of the problems that come from the adverse reactions, overuse, or misuse of medications among older people, but we do know, clearly, that it's an alarming situation that affects your health, your quality of life, and your pocketbook. As it is, older people currently account for nearly one-fourth of the health-care expenditures in this country. As a group, older people see doctors more often, go into hospitals more often, and once there, stay longer than people under the age of sixty-five. How many of your complaints and disabilities are actually *caused* by problems related to the drugs you take is difficult to determine. Drug-related problems are more difficult to detect, and sometimes harder to resolve than problems of disease. The consequences of drugs prescribed unnecessarily or in excessive doses can be seen in the exacerbation of illnesses and in otherwise unneeded visits to doctors, emergency rooms, hospitals, and other health-care facilities. The consequences can be seen in cases where prescribed drugs have caused Parkinson's disease or induced confusion, mental lapses, or fainting. Thousands of hip fractures and other broken bones—extremely serious in older people—are attributable to falls that result from dizziness or imbalance caused by medication. Sometimes, more often than we know, reactions to medications result in death.

Each year approximately sixty-one thousand older people develop drug-induced parkinsonism, and some thirty-two thousand have hip fractures as a result of drug-induced falls, according to Dr. Sidney Wolfe, M.D., his coauthors, and the Public Citizen Health Research Group in their recent book, *Worst Pills Best Pills*. They estimate that 163,000 older people have drug-induced or worsened memory loss or impaired thinking every year, and 243,000 are hospitalized yearly because of adverse reactions to medications.

It well may be that far more than 243,000 older people are admitted to hospitals because of adverse drug reactions, since so many medication reactions of older people are never detected, and rather are misdiagnosed as new problems. Researchers don't agree on the exact figures of drug-related hospital admissions, but according to Dr. Peter Lamy, a nationally known expert in geriatric pharmacology, between 12 and 17 percent of hospital admissions for people over the age of seventy are entirely due to adverse drug reactions. Dr. Lamy, director of the Center for the Study of Pharmacy and Therapeutics for the Elderly, and chairman of the Department of Pharmacy Practice at the University of Maryland at Baltimore, points out that these figures mean that one out of every six hospital admissions is caused by drugs. (That compares to only one in thirty to thirty-five hospital admissions for the entire population.) Dr. James Cooper at the University of Georgia College of Pharmacy, who conducted research in two different communities in Rhode Island and Idaho in the late 1970s, found that one out of every three hospital admissions was drug related. Dr. Cooper has also found that one out of every seven hospital admissions to nursing homes was drug related. In follow-up examinations, he found that four out of every five nursing home patients have significant drug-related problems.

Hidden Costs and Adverse Reactions
Dr. Helene Lipton, associate professor at the School of Pharmacy at the University of California at San Francisco, points out that there is a lack of good data on prescribing problems and how they can be solved more effectively. Many people take more or less medicine

than prescribed, or combine prescription drugs with nonprescription drugs their doctor doesn't know they're taking, which results in trips to emergency rooms, physicians' offices, or hospitals for undetected drug problems, she says. The full extent of the problem isn't known because there are no reliable studies that document drug-related incidents that aren't recognized by either doctor or patient. Many of them are treated as new diseases or are just assumed to be a worsening of the old disease.

"The saddest thing is when medicine causes a side effect and the physician believes it's a new disease for which you need a new drug," says Dr. Jerry Avorn, associate professor and director of the Programs for the Analysis of Clinical Strategies at Harvard Medical School.

Dr. Cooper found that in nine out of ten cases where there were drug-related problems, doctors were not aware that the problems of their patients *were* drug related; they thought the diseases were getting worse, not that the patients were having a reaction to their medication or were using the drug improperly. Another study said that patients more often than not didn't tell their physicians when they weren't taking the prescribed medication or were taking it intermittently. Because of these unknown quantities, it seems possible that drugs are playing an even larger role than we realize in the sicknesses of older people.

"You do have a real detection problem here," said Dr. Avorn. "If you don't know what's going on, you can't report it."

"We think, we don't know, we *think* that two to three percent of the older population dies from adverse drug reactions," says Dr. Lamy. "Is two or three percent relatively low? Yes. But is it unacceptable to the person to whom it happens? Absolutely! Particularly since most of those deaths are avoidable! We shouldn't have *any* adverse reactions!"

The Mysterious Symptom

One of the biggest indicators of how widespread the problems with medication are among the older population comes from Hugo Koch, a health statistician at the National Center for Health Statistics in Hyattsville, Maryland. Mr. Koch evaluated the drug data obtained in an extensive survey of medical care provided to older people by doctors in office-based practices. In his study of some 135 million prescriptions written in 1980 and 1981 for patients seventy-five and over, Mr. Koch inadvertently found that the main complaint patients had during their visit was dizziness. What was fascinating was that the dizziness had little correlation to the main physical condition for which the patients were being treated. Although sometimes ''dizziness'' can be a difficult complaint to diagnose because it can represent anything from sleepiness to anxiety to a funny feeling to light-headedness, it is a major symptom of the body's reaction to medications. Mr. Koch says he was led to the conclusion that the chief complaint that brought these patients to see their doctors was induced to an unknown degree by the use of medications—especially by their multiple use.

Simply put, this would mean that dizziness was caused by the side effects of medications, which may have been made worse by overdosage of medicines or multiple medications. **This means that the use of medicines—directly or indirectly—*is* a major cause of disability and illness among older people in this country.**

It's alarming to think that the substances you are relying on to make you feel better can actually induce further illness. As Napoleon said so long ago, ''I do not wish two diseases, one nature-made and one man-made''—but this unwanted wish comes true daily for many older Americans today.

Underuse a Problem

While overmedication and doses that are too large are a critical problem, those of you who need medications may sometimes be undermedicated. This is a serious problem that has rarely been examined. "The problems with undermedication are very important," says Dr. Lipton. "When people make decisions to discontinue antibiotics or to stop taking antihypertensive medications or antidepressants because they feel better, they can also get into real trouble. These issues haven't been examined thoroughly."

An indicator of the severity of undermedication can often be seen in the consequences of not taking cardiovascular medications that are needed. One review of studies related to cardiovascular disease and compliance with drug therapy estimated that 125,000 people die each year from *failure* to take their cardiovascular medicine as prescribed, most of them from taking too little or stopping the medication without follow-up. This figure is two and a half times the number of people killed yearly in car accidents and more than six times the number killed by firearms.

"I think of 'Edith Townsend,' who passed out because her potassium level was too low," "Stella Roth" said to me. "She fainted and was taken straight to the emergency room. She should have been on potassium, but she'd run out and just didn't bother to get any more of it. A couple of times when I've gone somewhere for three days and forgotten my potassium, I've been able to get what I needed from a pharmacist just to cover me! I don't want to go around fainting or putting that kind of stress on my body!"

Other patients with whom I talked also were aware that the dangers of not taking their medications consistently and properly were serious. "I just sent my sister a letter telling her what I'd heard about niacin, which she prescribes for herself," seventy-six-year-old "Margaret Landorf'' told me recently. "The report said that while niacin is a good thing for older people to take, it can be dangerous if not taken in the right amounts.

"I just open my ears trying to hear everything I can about medications," she said. "I do it because I want to have good health! It wouldn't be a convenient time for me to die!

"If I overdid it or got absentminded and didn't keep entirely alert, I know it could be a critical thing. I have five prescription medicines that I put out for myself every morning. I don't miss them. I know people who have died from not taking their medications—and people who have died from taking too many. They went overboard in one direction or another. It's easy to foul up your level of everything by not being consistent."

WHY DO WE HAVE A DRUG CRISIS?

The reasons for this enormous drug crisis are many and varied. Chief among them is that more drugs are available than ever before—and we don't know enough about them and their effects on older people. Given the phenomenon of modern medicine and modern drugs, it shouldn't be surprising to anyone that medicines have assumed a precarious and powerful role in our lives. Perhaps because they're so new and we're such trusting consumers of them, we take them either far too seriously (the cure is in a bottle of pills) or not nearly seriously enough ("Here, take one of my pressure pills, it'll help you feel better!").

Additionally, a great deal of the mismanagement in the medication of older Americans seems to happen because so little is known about healthy old age. That's not surprising when you consider how rapidly our older population has grown. The National Institute on Aging points out that in the past eighty-five years, we've gained *twenty-five years* in life expectancy—a gain that was duplicated only over the preceding five thousand years.

This momentous revolution has all happened so quickly that our society and the rest of the world are reeling from its social, medical, and economic implications. It's as if our newfound health has delivered us the kind of gift that people receive with gratitude, but hold uncertainly as they inspect it and think, "It looks good, but what do I do with it?" We feel we will benefit from "The Graying of Nations" and yet we still don't know quite how to respond to the many challenges presented us by such vast numbers of older people in the world.

We're already beginning to grapple with a number of issues—subsidized housing, medical services, public service needs, and long-term health insurance; revising Medicare, the federally financed health-insurance program that now pays for 45 percent of the health expenses for all older people (not including their prescriptions, dental care, glasses, hearing aids, or foot care), and Medicaid, which pays the balance of those health bills for the older poor who qualify. Medicaid is expected to skyrocket as the expanding population increases the number of people in nursing homes. We know we need to explore ways of reducing long-term health-care costs by creating community support services for ambulatory and home health care as alternatives to more expensive (and sometimes isolating) institutionalization. At the same time we need to increase social services—including mental health programs that meet the specific needs of the elderly—and effectively train the professionals and support personnel who will be needed to provide those services.

Our research needs are also great. Although we are learning more and more about the physiological effects of old age, we still don't know why aging bodies work the way they do—or even *how* they work for sure.

The Unknowns of Aging

Most of us first experience some aspects of our destiny when we watch our grandparents and parents getting older. What we see in them, and then begin to see in ourselves, constitutes our most intimate education in the process of aging.

If you are over sixty-five, or if you have older parents, you will have noticed changes taking place. We don't yet know all the mysteries of *why* these changes occur, but we do know *what* happens to us as we age. Most of us find ourselves experiencing certain physical declines: our eyesight changes; we hold the menu at arm's length in order to focus on the words; we need more light for reading. Our skin wrinkles and tends to change texture while our hair pales from black to white, from brown to gray, from red to blond or brown. Our circulation, hearing, joints, and energy levels behave differently. Even when we're marathon runners, we can't run as fast; we can't do as many push-ups. Many of us acquire chronic health problems and have a greater need for medical intervention than we did when we were younger. B.F. Skinner said there was no denying that as we grow older, our senses become less acute and our muscles weaker. "Someone has said that if you want to know what it feels like to be old," Skinner wrote in his book *Enjoy Old Age*, "you should smear dirt on your glasses, stuff cotton in your ears, put on heavy shoes that are too big for you, and wear gloves; then try to spend the day in a normal way."

We are learning that the process of aging is a complex and highly individualized happening. Up until recently, most of the data physicians, scientists, and health-care professionals have collected on older people has come from nursing-home and hospital patients—not from older adults who live in the community. Therefore, the studies medical students, osteopaths, nurses, and pharmacists have read about older people for the most part were based on studies from sick older people, not healthy ones. This has drastically affected what is known about normal aging and the effects of medicines on older people—and is key to many of today's drug misuse problems. When it comes to aging and medicine, lack of information about the subject is the rule, not the exception.

"The medicine of old age is not the medicine of young people," says Dr. John W. Rowe, former director of the Division on Aging at the Harvard Medical School. "Our view of healthy aging is based largely on disease. A main task of gerontology today is the effort to differentiate disease from the process of aging. We simply don't know about normal aging."

The Unknowns of Pharmacology

Similarly, we don't know about aging and its interaction with medicines. Just as this is the "first century of old age," it is also, in many ways, the first century of pharmacology.

When I first interviewed Dr. Bernard Mehl in the pharmacy department at Mount Sinai Medical Center in New York, I said that I understood that pharmacology had only been an "exact science" for some thirty years. Dr. Mehl laughed.

"It's questionable that it's an 'exact science' even now," he said. "Determining the appropriate dosage is difficult. It's very difficult to say that a given dose is exactly what any patient will need. There are many variables that can result in side effects or lack of an effect. The amount of the drug you have to give has to be accurate to avoid reaching a toxic level, yet that amount can vary because of weight, sex, and age and other factors you have to consider.

"Pharmacology is experimental in the sense that a doctor will prescribe a drug and then has to carefully observe what effects there are. He has to make sure there are no adverse reactions, and he also has to watch to see that the drug is doing what it's supposed to do."

Because there are so many thousands of medicines, and because so many of them have played such a large role in medical treatment in the recent past, it's hard to remember that the explosive increase in medicines is a post–World War II phenomenon. While there have been some pretty good medicines available for a long time, there are many more drugs now, as well as a bigger selection within each category defined as appropriate therapy for different diseases. Hundreds of drugs are quite new—and so is our understanding of the ways they work within the body.

The pharmaceutical industry, one of the biggest, most profitable enterprises in America, continues to research and manufacture new drugs that are more effective, more powerful, and more costly to customers. (One arthritis preparation alone, Feldene, brings in more than $600 million a year for Pfizer Drug Corporation.) Large pharmaceutical companies pour $100 million into the development of each new drug, and many of those drugs never even reach the market. The drugs that go nowhere are referred to as "black holes" by the drug industry. The ones that do hit the market survive stringent quality control tests to meet licensing requirements for safety and effectiveness from the Federal Food and Drug Administration (FDA).

It's not like the days when the medicine man sold three varieties of snake oil from the back of his wagon. It's not even like it was when most medicines didn't work very well or the side effects outweighed their effectiveness—when the best therapy physicians could offer was compassion and a positive outlook. Today the pharmaceutical companies advertise their carefully controlled and inspected substances directly to doctors, who in turn have the authority to write prescriptions for their patients. Although physicians tend to stick primarily to popular drugs, they have a wide variety to choose from. In 1991, there were 10,003 FDA-approved prescription drugs on the market. That doesn't count drugs that predate licensing laws, like morphine, or reserpine, which is so ancient that it was first written about in Sanskrit. By the time you add in all the old, unregistered drugs, the new generic drugs, and all the registered drugs available in all their forms and dosages, a spokesman for the Pharmaceutical Manufacturers Association says it's not an exaggeration to say there are about 100,000 prescription drugs currently on the market. (This does not count the 300,000 over-the-counter medications the Non-Prescription Drug Manufacturers Association says it has on the market.)

The licensing requirements and big money involved still don't provide us with all the answers we want about these drugs. Despite the high standards of pharmaceutical companies, it's often impossible to be sure of a drug's long-term, or even short-term, effects with the functioning of a particular patient's body.

The Unknowns of Geriatric Pharmacology

Because increasing numbers of older people are taking increasing numbers of drugs, we could say that this is also the "first century of geriatric pharmacology." Until recently, drugs weren't manufactured, tested, or monitored with the unique problems of older people in mind. Even today, standard dosages of most drugs used by all ages are tested mainly on healthy people in their twenties and thirties, not on people in their seventies, eighties, or nineties—so most drug labels and manuals don't specify recommended dosages for older people. Recently, however, the FDA issued guidelines encouraging manufacturers to test their drugs on a wider range of the population and to conduct research that would indicate how drugs are metabolized in older people as well as in younger people so that information could be included in labeling. Although these guidelines are suggestions, not requirements, the pharmaceutical industry has begun to pay closer attention to drugs used primarily by older people, and a number of companies have taken steps to test drugs on older people and publicize their results. So far, however, there are no mandatory specifications that drugs be tested on older people.

To meet FDA approval, the premarketing studies involve one thousand people in a control group and one thousand people in an active drug group. "This is enough people to answer the question of whether a drug is effective and to see its common side effects," says New York internist Dr. Barbara Otto, "but disastrous side effects are rare—sometimes as few as one in ten thousand cases—so the required sample of people means there's a good chance of missing adverse reactions completely." As a result, it's only *after* a drug has been on the market for a number of years that its full therapeutic—and harmful—potential can be determined. Even then, the full range of possible effects is often not documented or known. Once a drug has been approved by the FDA for sale and is on the market, there is no mandatory follow-up of that drug. Prescribing physicians and patients may or may not make voluntary reports of problems and side effects to the drug manufacturer or the FDA. Any follow-up to the FDA is entirely dependent on the individual physician who has the motivation or feels it's incumbent on him to pinpoint specific side effects of the drug. (A doctor, for instance, who sees that a new anti-inflammatory drug is causing renal failure and death, should report that information to the FDA. But he may or may not do so.) A vast number of adverse drug reactions go unreported and uncorrected.

"The concept [of having drugs tested in the elderly] has met with resistance because it's more expensive," says Dr. Bernard Mehl at Mount Sinai Medical Center in New York City. "But you have a lot more older people, a lot more drugs, and a lot more recognition that there are differences. We didn't have that awareness before. Now that there's that recognition, now that there are going to be a lot more older people—and they're going to be us—there has to be the testing. No matter what difficulties are involved, it should be done.''

"The FDA gives approval for the use of drugs for people over the age of thirteen," says Dr. Otto. "This gives a special recognition to the dangers of drug dosages for young children because of their size. Different sizes means different requirements in dosing. And certainly older people require varying doses depending on their size and a number of other factors. Maybe the FDA warning should say, 'This drug has not been tested on people sixty-five and older,' which would give special recognition to the dangers to older people. Also, the FDA should set up an active reporting system of trying to follow the use of new drugs in people sixty-five and older. If physicians were *required* to report to the FDA on the use of drugs, at least in the case of a person who has an adverse reaction, the information could be used to help others.''

What People Don't Know About Their Medications
Many of the hazardous results of drug misuse could be avoided if we understood more about the risks involved in our use of medications, and more about managing them.

"A major problem that makes the use and effectiveness of drugs even more unpredictable is that patients are unreliable about cooperating with the prescription," says Dr. Mehl, who points out that doctors often don't know whether or not their patients are taking their prescribed drugs as directed. "Patients have to cooperate in order for doctors to determine whether the drug is or is not effective," he says. "Doctors are dependent on their patients for this information.''

Apparently, many patients could do a much better job than they do of reporting back to their doctors on what they've done with the prescriptions they've been given. For a variety of reasons, however, a large number of people simply don't take their medications as directed. For instance, studies have shown that:

- Over half of people over sixty-five don't take their prescriptions as directed.
- Patients don't tell their doctors what other drugs, including over-the-counter drugs, they're taking.
- Patients don't know the name of the drug prescribed, don't know how to use it, and don't know why they're taking it.
- About 10 percent don't get prescriptions filled in the first place due to the expense involved, because they feel better, or decide to use something else instead.
- Patients often swap medicines with friends and make other decisions about medications without consulting their doctors.

Patients report that they leave the doctor's office, the clinic, and the pharmacy with no information on the drugs' side effects and no special instructions on how to take the medicines. Why does this happen? Some clues come from studies that document the time doctors spend talking to their patients about prescriptions. One study established that doctors spent one minute giving information about drugs to their patients.

Referring to the report of a Harris Poll that found that doctors spent an average of two to six minutes talking with their patients about as many as four different drugs, Joe Graedon, author of *The New People's Pharmacy*, pointed out, "That's hardly enough time to pronounce the name of some of the drugs, let alone give instructions for their use or warnings about possible problems and interactions."

"He gave me something for my viral infection," "Joe Smithers" told his wife, Sally, when he got home from an evening visit to a new doctor in Boca Raton, Florida. "I guess it's antibiotics. There's also this cough syrup."

"Are you supposed to take the pills with meals or before meals or what?" Sally asked.

"I don't know."

"Why don't you know?!" she demanded. "Didn't you ask him?"

"The whole visit was about five minutes," Joe explained. "He just walked in and looked up from the chart and said, 'I'm Dr. Walters.' He didn't ask me my name or anything. I barely had time to tell him how I was feeling. I thought of all kinds of questions after I was out of his office."

Even when doctors do talk to their patients about their prescriptions, the patients often don't understand what is being said. Dr. Bonnie Svarstadt, a professor of Social Behavior and Pharmacy at the School of Pharmacy at the University of Wisconsin, observed patient visits at a neighborhood health center in the Bronx in the early '70s. There, she observed that more than three out of four times, the physician failed to give explicit instructions about how regularly or how often drugs should be taken. When the physicians did give instructions, Dr. Svarstadt herself often found those instructions confusing, incomplete, or ambiguous.

Subsequent studies have confirmed Dr. Svarstadt's observations. Unclear instructions seem to be the rule, not the exception, when it comes to doctor-patient communication. For instance, if you are told to take one pill a day, should you take it in the morning or in the evening? Should you take it with food, before food, or after food? Does one tablet every six hours mean that you should wake up in the middle of your sleep to take the fourth tablet or does it mean that you should only take these pills when you're awake—which would mean three a day?

Geriatric nurses observe that many of their patients don't realize that there are certain foods or beverages they should or should not take with their medicines. They're not given a basic understanding about the purpose of the prescription. In Dr. Svarstadt's study, more than half of the people she interviewed misunderstood why they were taking their drugs in the first place. Patients who had been given medications for high blood pressure sometimes thought their prescriptions were for symptoms such as asthma or lower back pain. From numerous interviews and studies, it seems clear that patients aren't being told basic information about their prescriptions. Most doctors don't tell you, for instance, that you need this particular drug to keep you from having a stroke or to cure an infection, and that you need to use the drug regularly. You're not told in some critical cases that this drug might make you feel worse temporarily, but that you should take it anyway because if you don't you might possibly have eye damage or heart damage.

The Communication Gap

"Drug misuse happens because no one has taken the time to educate people about their medicines," says Dr. Cooper at the University of Georgia. "They've either been too timid or too accepting to know they have the right to ask."

Odds are that better communication would make a big dent in the numbers of people entering hospitals because of problems caused by their medications. And while many studies have been conducted on how patients don't comply with their drug regime, little has been done on how to improve that compliance. Studies have shown, however, that in general one-on-one discussion changes behavior better than written communication does. It would seem to follow that when doctors are open to what you have to say—when they allow you to tell your story in your own words and to comment on suggestions—compliance with instructions would improve. Another reason that one-on-one discussion would seem to work more effectively is that it uses more of your senses and involves you more thoroughly—thus more effectively changing behavior. Written information in addition to the verbal information could make a substantial difference in proper use and administration of drugs and perhaps save millions of dollars in health care expenditures every year.

Physician Reticence

"Sometimes physicians are opposed to written information about drugs being disseminated because they're nervous about the prospect of patients finding out about a side effect they didn't tell them about and coming back and saying, 'Why did you give me a prescription that would make me such and such?,' " says Dr. Jerry Avorn at Harvard Medical School. "Physicians are also concerned that if patients read about side effects, they might develop them," he said. "They also state a fear that if the patient reads about the side effects, it might reduce compliance." Dr. Avorn pointed out, however, that a lengthy study commissioned by the FDA and administered by the Rand Corporation showed that many of the bugaboos cited as potential problems simply are not real. Evidence from that study showed that there was no difference in the development of symptoms between a group of patients who were totally informed about the side effects of their drugs and a similar group who weren't informed about side effects. Other studies have confirmed that giving people more information does not produce more symptoms.

"Basically, physicians' reluctance to share this kind of information is part of their historic inability to educate their patients," said Dr. Avorn. "When the patients have information about their medications, many physicians feel on the defensive. They want to keep the entire flow of information under their control. It's the old concept of physician as God the Father—that is, patients should do what we tell them to do. It's been going on for thousands of years. Even with the shamans and healers there was an air of mystery about what they used in their healing process. That's the mysterious part of prescribing. When patients have information about their medications, it means they're looking behind the mask. It takes away the magic. Yet it seems clear to me that physicians today should use drugs because they work pharmacologically, not by magic.''

More and more, the mystique of pharmacology is being invaded by consumers. The first step in resolving—and preventing—problems with drugs is learning what you need to know. A recent poll by CBS TV and CBS Economics reported that more than one-third of the households they polled used *The Physicians' Desk Reference* for information about prescription drugs. More than two-thirds said they considered information on blood pressure, heart problems, and life-threatening diseases to be highly important. Many others I talked with use James Long's *The Essential Guide to Prescription Drugs* and *The Merck Manual* whenever they get a new prescription. Yet it's clear that the information from these sources still isn't enough. It doesn't reach enough people and may not always have an impact when it does. Slightly more than three-fourths of the people polled by CBS said they felt only ''somewhat informed'' or ''not informed at all.''

Other avenues of information, however, are opening up. The American Association of Retired Persons (AARP) now publishes and distributes medical brochures to their members and anyone who requests them. The leaflets, Medication Information Leaflets for Seniors (MILS), are geared specifically to the geriatric population. They name the class of medication, tell what it's for, how to take it, how long to take it, and its possible side effects. With nitroglycerin, for instance, the MILS will tell you that the effects of the drug will be faster depending on the route of the drug— i.e., whether you are taking a tablet, using a nitropatch, or taking it sublingually (under the tongue). The MILS also remind you what your doctor should know about you before you take the medication. These leaflets are written in large type and are available at no cost through the AARP Pharmacy Service (510 King Street, Alexandria, Virginia 22314), the largest private pharmaceutical mail service in the country.

The National Council on Patient Information and Education (NICPIE) has launched a nationwide educational program on patient use and misuse of medications, as has Parke-Davis, with a program called Elder-Care. Modeled after the Elder-Health Program at the University of Maryland School of Pharmacy, Elder-Care is a national consumer drug education program for older people, their families, and care-givers. Practicing pharmacists, faculty, and pharmacy students present programs in forty-five states at senior centers and schools to discuss issues related to medications and their management. Elder-Care also mails out free brochures with advice on managing medications. (Elder-Care, 201 Tabor Rd., Morris Plains, N.J. 09750.)

The American Medical Association (AMA) has also prepared one-page patient medication instruction sheets (PMI) on 250 of the most commonly prescribed drugs. Each PMI describes the purpose of the drug, how it is to be taken, its possible side effects, and what the patient should tell the doctor. These sheets are available for your doctor to order and to give to you. Doctors and pharmacists can also order and give you Patient Advisory Leaflets (PALS) from Pharmex Professional Review Committee, which consists of physicians and pharmacists (Pharmex, A Division of Automatic Business Products Co., Inc., PO Box 57, Willimantic, Connecticut 06226). These leaflets describe the purpose of the medicine, how to take it, precautions, side effects, and general instructions for safe use.

The National Cancer Institute's hotline (1-800-4-CANCER) and the information network sponsored by the American Cancer Society (1-800-ACS-2345) both provide up-to-date information about cancer and cancer treatment for patients and family members. Questions about the purpose, administration, and side effects of cancer drugs, chemotherapy, radiation, and the most current treatments for various cancers are answered thoroughly and carefully. Respondents sitting at computer terminals have the latest information at their fingertips. This is an excellent (and free) resource that can help you cope with questions and concerns about cancer.

GERIATRICS—A STEP IN THE RIGHT DIRECTION

Even the most knowledgeable physicians are hard pressed to keep up with the massive amount of information on the thousands and thousands of today's drugs, their side effects, and their interaction with other drugs. Additionally, most physicians lack training in gerontology or geriatrics. (Gerontology, by the way, is the study of many aspects of aging, from biological investigations at the molecular level to socioeconomic investigations into the effect of such things as bereavement or retirement on health and social status. Geriatrics refers to a wide scope of clinical studies of the diseases, disabilities, and health of older people. A subspecialty of internal medicine or family practice, geriatrics merges information from gerontology, neurology, psychiatry, urology, orthopedics, social work, and pharmacology.) A physician who has been trained in geriatrics will realize that he sees different manifestations of the same disease in older and in younger people. He'll know that a younger person with an overactive thyroid is usually jittery and overactive, while an older person suffering from the same condition will often be slow, lethargic, and depressed. He'll also recognize that pain thresholds change as we age, too. An older person who's having an acute appendicitis attack may only have a sore throat, whereas a younger person would be doubled over in pain. Too often, doctors who haven't been trained in geriatrics have failed to recognize the seriousness of such symptoms.

"My father died because the weekend doctor didn't realize he had pneumonia," says "Trudy Vandenhovel," who lives in a suburb of Philadelphia. "He had a high fever and no pain, not even a headache. His body was very stiff with Parkinson's, but the doctor could not find anything special. He said it wasn't serious, it was probably a flu, and that we should give him liquids and bathe him to keep the fever down. By the time his own doctor came to see him, he was very very sick. He could hardly speak and hardly use his body. He was delirious and restless. The doctor said he had to go to the hospital immediately to find out what was wrong. Two hours after we got to the hospital, he died. The doctor said he had died from pneumonia. They hadn't diagnosed him soon enough to save him."

Dr. Robert Butler points out that when the present generation of medical-school graduates reaches the prime of their careers, approximately 60 percent of their work will involve geriatrics. "I like to counsel medical students that if you're not interested in older people," he says, "then you've got one choice, and that's to go into pediatrics or to give up medicine entirely. Because the name of the game is going to be older persons."

The rapid growth in the older population has greatly increased the demand for formal training of medical students in geriatrics. In 1988, however, only 13 of the 126 medical schools in the United States *required* their medical students to take courses or clinical rotations in geriatrics. And during that same year, according to the American Association of Medical Colleges, only 3.5 percent of medical-school graduates had taken a course in geriatrics during all of medical school. Clinical programs that give medical students practical experience dealing with older people still don't exist in many departments of internal medicine or departments of family practice.

Currently, of the 600,780 practicing physicians in this country, only 1,153 list their primary specialty as geriatrics, according to the 1991 records from the Physician Data Service of the American Medical Association.

While the National Institute on Aging is funding fellowships in geriatrics, and urging others to do the same, geriatric training is still embryonic in the majority of medical schools. As recently as the mid 1970s, many doctors who wanted to specialize in geriatrics traveled abroad for training. Since 1980, the training of geriatricians to practice medicine, to teach, and to pursue basic and clinical research, has accelerated in medical schools across the country. In schools that have traditionally emphasized geriatrics, such as New York University, Boston University, the University of Michigan, Duke University, Johns Hopkins, UCLA, and the University of Southern California, medical divisions of geriatrics have been strengthened. In 1982, the Mount Sinai School of Medicine established a department of geriatrics and adult development, and made a geriatrics rotation for fourth-year students a requirement. In a 1986 survey, Dr. Edward L. Schneider, then deputy director of the National Institute on Aging, found that at least 80 percent of the academic medical centers in the country included clinical programs to give medical students practical experience in geriatrics and long-term care.

Even with this increased emphasis, however, the number throughout the United States of part-time or full-time geriatrics faculty who teach all levels of undergraduates, residents, and midcareer positions ranges from a nationwide high of 909 in internal medicine to a low of 86 in physical medicine and rehabilitation. Tables developed by the Rand Corporation indicate that we will need close to two thousand faculty members

teaching geriatrics to meet the health-care needs of the
elderly by the year 2000.

"We need to see that all practicing physicians have
training in geriatrics because it will be a component of
the practice of medicine in virtually all fields of medicine, with the exception of pediatrics," says Dr. T.
Franklin Williams, director of the National Institute on
Aging. "To accomplish that, we need more teachers
and academic leaders."

In an effort to further encourage practicing physicians
to focus on geriatric issues, the American Board of
Family Practice and the American Board of Internal
Medicine have offered special examinations to determine competence in geriatric medicine. Beginning in
1988, courses in geriatrics have been given across the
country to prepare physicians for this special certifica-
tion procedure. So far, 4,085 physicians certified in
family medicine or internal medicine have been awarded
certificates of added qualification in geriatrics. Examinations scheduled for 1992 and 1994 should increase
that number. Additionally, the Merck Foundation and
other drug companies are supporting fellowships in geriatrics and in geriatric clinical pharmacology in an effort
to encourage more doctors to focus on the problems of
drugs and the elderly. Based on current levels of entry
into geriatrics, some 6,970 internists and family physicians will be certified in geriatrics by the year 2000,
according to Dr. John C. Beck, director of the Multi-
campus Division of Geriatrics and Gerontology at
UCLA, who conducted a recent study for the Bureau
of Health Professions in the Health Resources and Services Administration in Washington, D.C.

Pharmacists and nurses are also attempting to close
the gaps in their training of students who will be dealing
with the health-care problems of the elderly.

"Geriatrics used to be covered in pharmacy curricula
as part of other disciplines such as pharmacology or
therapeutics, but it wasn't recognized as a specific dis-

cipline until the last five years," says Richard Penna, associate executive director of the American Association of Colleges of Pharmacy (AACP). "Now at least three pharmacy schools have developed certificates in geriatric therapeutics based on a complete curriculum." According to Jacqueline Eng at the AACP, sixty of the some seventy-three colleges of pharmacy are now planning to institute a geriatric curriculum into their academic program within the next year. The same curriculum is being used by many nursing schools.

Nurses, who usually have the most intimate contact with patients and their medications, have always focused more on geriatrics than their colleagues have. Their training and their clinical experience with older people far surpasses similar training for doctors or pharmacists. In a survey of 220 schools of nursing, the American Association of Colleges of Nursing found in 1985 that 91 percent of the respondent schools included gerontological nursing in their baccalaureate curricula. "I would assume that nearly one hundred percent of our nurses are exposed to the clinical courses with a nursing component in geriatrics," says Judith M. Cassells, R.N., D.N.Sc., project director of AACN. "There's room for stronger emphasis in geriatrics in the theoretical and clinical content in all our courses, however, and room for more required separate course work as well."

GETTING TO THE HEART OF THE PROBLEM

Modern medicine and pharmacology involve elaborate systems of specialized, technical knowledge and skill. Sometimes, when I hear horror stories of older patients stumbling and breaking bones because of being groggy from overmedication, when I hear that a vigorous seventy-year-old man went into heart failure because a doctor at the hospital didn't check his chart before prescribing a drug that was lethal, my knee-jerk reaction is to agree with the view of social critic Ivan Illich that medical care causes more disease than it cures. I realize, however, that both doctors and patients make mistakes. Even when a physician is 100 percent on target about a prescription she writes for her patient, the patient can sabotage treatment by forgetting a dose and later taking two to make up for the forgotten one. Sometimes the patient slips off to a second doctor, gets a second (or third) prescription, and never tells either doctor about all the drugs. Sometimes even when the doctor and patient have behaved impeccably, the drug itself or the unique nature of a body are at fault. Drugs can inexplicably go haywire within a particular person's body or they adversely interact with other chemical conditions within the body, with another drug, with food, alcohol, or with another disease. The unpredictability of many variables prevents a simple explanation.

Advocate on Your Own Behalf

The bottom line is that *you* must be vigilant. Certainly diseases are more specifically defined than they used to be, and doctors have a great deal of knowledge available to help them analyze your medical history and to make their diagnosis. The high-powered diagnostic tools and lab reports they use to confirm or contradict their diagnosis can sometimes supersede the need for brilliance on the doctor's part or your part. Nevertheless, *you* are the main source of information about your condition. The history you give the doctor will determine what he prescribes for you. His diagnosis depends on that history. After the diagnosis is made and confirmed, you should still be involved. How you deal with your condition, how crippling your treatment might be, and what risks are involved are matters that should always concern you. By now you should be well aware that if you don't have your own interest in mind, you can't expect that someone else will. A lot is still unknown about drugs, but one of the best ways to make sure they help, not harm, you is to know all you can about them, about your own health, and about the way your body works.

Old age can be an invigorating and productive time of life. If you plan to keep functioning in good spirits and comfortable circumstances, it's reassuring to know that you probably can. You can trust that when health problems arise, medications can be very useful. When they're carefully prescribed, followed, and monitored by both patient and doctor, they can get you through sicknesses, keep your body chemistry balanced, and stave off what otherwise might be crippling diseases. They can also relieve subtle discomforts and enhance your feeling of well-being.

If you're older, or if you have older parents dependent on you, remember that you can't afford to avoid responsibility when it comes to taking medicine; it must be a shared responsibility. Every person is a unique system, and no one knows it better than the person whose body it is. As Alice Green said, "Why, I can't imagine why people ask the doctor to tell them how they feel. *I* know how I feel! When I see the doctor, I tell him—he doesn't tell me!"

The more you know about what to expect of yourself as you age, and the more you expect to feel good, vital, and healthy, the more you'll be able to use medications effectively. There are no hard-and-fast rules. Older people are pioneers in this business—and just like any other pioneers, your survival depends on astute observation, responsiveness, and action. You can understand your own body by observing changes in it, by learning what to expect, and by sharing clues and information about changes, especially when your ability to live your life fully is affected in any negative way.

For your own protection, keep in mind that, just like your doctor, you may not always know the difference between being sick and being old.

"He gave me these little red pills to help my heart," sixty-eight-year-old "Harriet Engel" told me one afternoon when we were talking about her medical history. "They made me throw up every morning and get dizzy every afternoon."

"Didn't you tell the doctor?"

"Well, I thought I'd get used to them, but I didn't," she said. "I told him when I had my next appointment. He said he'd cut it down a bit, and when he did, that made a big difference."

Mrs. Engel's reaction is typical. Because she accepts the view that she's supposed to feel different than she used to, she doesn't take proper care of herself or call on the help that's available to her.

If you live to be a hundred, there's no real reason why you shouldn't anticipate feeling good most of that time. Dr. Robert Butler tells the story of a 104-year-old who went to his doctor and complained that he had a pain in his left leg. The doctor asked him, "Well, what do you expect at your age?" The centurian said, "I expect my left leg to feel as good as my right leg! That's what I expect!"

CHAPTER 2

Am I Sick or Am I Just Getting Old?

Clara Glotzbach, a month away from her ninety-ninth birthday, sat talking with her ninety-three-year-old friend, Ida. Her large, lively eyes didn't seem to miss anything going on in the senior center, where the two old buddies had met to have lunch and play cards.

Clara, her white hair shining, wore a blue paisley dress with a lacy white collar. Before walking to the center from her home, she had baked a sweet-potato casserole to contribute to the potluck lunch.

For more than forty years, Clara lived with her husband on a farm outside Saint Mary's, Kansas, a small community that lies between Manhattan and Topeka. They had seven children. Now, in addition to her six living children and their spouses, she also has seven grandchildren and thirteen great-grandchildren.

"I'm hard of hearing and my eyes aren't very good, but I guess I can expect that at my age," she said, chuckling. "I take a little heart pill in the morning for my circulation, and some vitamins. I used to have phlebitis in my leg, but I took a lot of exercise and done a lot of walking, and it don't bother me anymore. I've taken the little heart pill since I was fifty years old. I was supposed to take 'em four times a day, but I don't."

The first time Clara ever went into the hospital was when she had just turned ninety-eight. She had a gallbladder infection and stayed in the hospital for two days. After that, she also spent one day (no overnight) in the hospital for eye surgery.

"I try to walk four blocks a day, and I use a cane," she said. "I did fall here the other day. I lost my balance when I leaned over to pick up a little piece of paper off the floor. When I use my cane, I still walk pretty good."

After I met Clara, I knew that George Bernard Shaw was right when he said, "Your legs give in before your head does."

A major obstacle to getting good health care is the myth that getting older means that you never feel well. Because so many of us—doctors and patients alike—have negative conceptions of what aging means, we equate getting older with feeling lousy. When we experience new aches, pains, or physical discomforts, we assume they're part of the package that comes with age, instead of treating them as symptoms of something gone wrong, as we did when we were younger. As a result, we often don't take care of serious physical problems that need attention.

Many older people I talked with told me they'd had problems that could have been nipped in the bud if they hadn't ignored, or adapted to, warning pains or discomforts. Because they thought the particular pain was "to be expected" as part of getting older, they delayed telling their doctors about symptoms they should have reported immediately.

"I was fooled," said Homer Arena, a retired pharmacist in New Jersey. "I had a pain in the side of my face, and I thought maybe I had a little infection. It was like the beginning of a toothache or swollen glands, just a dull ache. I had it three or four days and I didn't pay much attention to it. I just took an aspirin at night, but the pain woke me up. Still I didn't pay any attention. I should have known better and gone for treatment, but I didn't. I ended up with chest pains and a heart attack. Now I know that pain indicates that something is wrong and you'd better look into it.''

Mr. Arena's pain continued for a few days before his heart attack, which could have been deferred if treated. Some people go for months or years with symptoms that should have taken them to the doctor.

''I couldn't get him to go to the doctor,'' Norma Lepore said, looking at her husband, Dominick. ''He passed out on me for years, and he'd get all white and sweaty, but he'd never let me call the doctor. One time when he passed out in the bedroom and I tried to pick him up, I hit his head on the bedpost and cut his eye.''

Dominick Lepore, at sixty-six, sat back in his chair at the dinner table and ran his hand through the white chest hair peeking out from his open shirt. His fingers grazed a smooth, pearly-looking sliver of a scar that ran from beneath the dip at the base of his neck down his chest at an angle.

''What ever got you to go?'' I asked, studying the scar, wondering how long it had taken to heal.

''I started feeling different,'' he said, touching his neck. ''I started having this pulsing in here, and I figured it was probably more than just running out of steam. Before, I always figured it was just something that came with the territory, and I didn't want to let it get me down!''

''He never decided for himself to go,'' Norma protested. ''I made him go.''

Whatever, Dominick got there just in time. During his stress test, he passed out. Three days later he had a quadruple bypass.

Now, Dominick is back in good health. For a ''continuation of the heart operation,'' as he sees it, he now takes three aspirins and one digitalis tablet every day.

"I see the medicine as a necessary evil," he says. "That's why I do it."

Dominick Lepore was lucky. Because he finally got over his fear that he was "just getting old" and gave up on his macho insistence that "nothing was wrong," he's still alive today. He was able to have surgery and begin medication that decreases further risk of cardiac problems.

Some people aren't so lucky. Many people fail to report serious symptoms to the doctor because they think they're only "running out of steam," and by the time they do go, it's too late. Because there aren't a lot of rewards for getting old in our society, and because aging is often seen as a loss of status and vigor, growing older can create a great deal of internal ambivalence and conflict. The denial of what one considers the symptoms of aging, then, can become a way of denying the reality of getting older.

Some people also experience an undefined sense of shame about getting older that's fed by an unconscious association of "old" with "bad" or "feeble." They also may feel ashamed that their bodies aren't functioning properly, or that they're poor or not eating well. Shame makes them hide their pains and their embarrassment. Men, even more than women, seem to hate admitting to sickness or lack of well-being, because they equate it with weakness. They're "too proud" to show that weakness. Women often withhold information about serious illnesses because they don't want to be seen as "complaining old women" or "hypochondriacs." Sometimes, too, they're reticent about being seen as less attractive than they used to be. "I'm not showing this wrinkled old body to nobody," a feisty old woman outside a senior center declared to me one sunny afternoon. "Not the doctor or nobody! I'm even going to tell the funeral director to shut his eyes!"

Another reason older people don't go to the doctor when they should is that they're afraid of what the pain may indicate. Putting off the possibility of treating a condition, however, can lead to the kind of crisis or terminal situation that was feared in the first place.

PERSISTENT STEREOTYPES

Most stereotypes about aging are based on illnesses that in time may be reduced or altogether eliminated.

"Much of what we think of as aging today is actually disease and illness, and not a part of fundamental physical aging," says Dr. Robert N. Butler, sitting in his office in the geriatrics department at Mount Sinai School of Medicine. "In time, the major diseases of late life may become preventable or at least treatable. The mental depressions of late life and the acute brain syndromes are already treatable and reversible."

Until more is known, you might as well assume that there's no reason why you shouldn't feel good. Aching, feeling worn out, or having pain is *not* a necessary part of aging. If you quietly accept the discomforts without reporting them to the doctor, you may find out, too late, that your health problems could have been reversed or treated instead of requiring dramatic intervention or hospitalization at an advanced stage.

Sometimes, even when *you* know something is wrong, your doctor may tell you that it's just because you're "getting old." I talked with dozens of people who told me about going to see their doctors because they had some disquieting symptom, only to be told that they should "expect" to feel that way as they aged. Clearly, these doctors have not been trained in geriatrics. They're responding to stereotypes about aging based on the pathologies of older age—and they are uninformed about the realities of healthy aging.

"We need to clearly understand how a normal old person ages and how that differs from a normal younger person," says Dr. John W. Rowe, who directed Har-

vard Medical School's Division on Aging before becoming president of the Mount Sinai Medical Center in
New York. "Up until now, doctors and nurses compared a sick old person to a healthy young one. We still
know very little about the difference between a healthy
older person and a healthy younger person."

"Paul Lewis," a retired anthropology professor,
seemed to have his own notions about the difference
between being "old and healthy" and "old and sick."
His story is unusual only in that he was persistent in
his efforts to get a proper medical response. At the age
of eighty-one, Paul, who lived in Boise, Idaho, found
that he was tired all the time and sweating heavily in
the evenings for some weeks. "At each visit, I told my
doctor I was aging too fast," Paul said. "His answer
was, 'You've got to expect it.' Two or three months ago,
I decided that was an unsatisfactory answer, so I
switched doctors to a younger man. When I told him
that I was tired all the time and that it was getting worse,
he said, 'I'll see if we can find what's causing it.' "

The doctor put him through a series of tests and found
that Paul was anemic and that his heart was greatly
enlarged. When the doctor saw Paul's blood count drop
fifteen more points in the next two days, he told him
he thought he was suffering from gastrointestinal bleeding and needed to check into the hospital for a blood
transfusion. After three days and three transfusions,
Paul was released, feeling like a new man. "For the
first time in years, I was using my full chest capacity
in breathing," he said. "My saliva flowed again, and
my appetite returned. Even after being in bed for almost
four days, I felt stronger than I had in many months."

Older women, even more than men, often fall victim
to the physician's stereotypes about them, says gerontologist Myrna Lewis, who is coauthor with Robert Butler of *Sex After Forty*. "If an older woman goes to see
a doctor, she is likely to be given a Valium," says Ms.
Lewis, "but if an older man goes in, he's given a com-

plete physical and possibly a CAT scan as well. Doctors just take the complaints of men more seriously than they take the complaints of women.''

Some doctors tend to see a woman's physical complaints as emotionally related, says Ms. Lewis, and as a result they don't do the kind of thorough diagnostic work necessary to make a proper determination of the case. Although some complaints are in fact related to life events that cause depression and resulting lethargy, they all deserve to be properly evaluated and treated.

''Andrea Diehl'' was one of several older women who told me about poor physician treatment. She had had a hiatus hernia for nearly three years before she found out what was causing her pain. When she told her family doctor about the pain, he insisted that it was ''just in her head,'' that she was having a reaction to retirement, and that it would pass. He patted her head and told her to take aspirin if she really thought she needed it. Not knowing better, she believed him and thought she just had to live with the pain. When her daughter-in-law finally got her to go to a different doctor for an examination, she learned that she needed immediate surgery for the hernia.

Beulah Kellogg had arthritis and a spur along her spinal column. Yet, despite her pain and the lack of an inquiring concern on the part of her doctor, Beulah never questioned her doctor's wisdom when he told her it was all a part of aging. As a farmer's wife in a rural area, she'd always lived far from good health-care facilities and hadn't had much experience with doctors. She was used to putting up with discomforts and adjusting herself to changes beyond her control. Not realizing that she was entitled to be relieved of her pain, she also simply didn't know what was—and what was not—natural to the process of aging.

Another stereotyped response older people report is that when they have one debilitating feature, people assume that they have broken down in other ways as well.

A person who moves about in a wheelchair, for instance, is often ignored—as if he were the chair, not the person. Many people who have difficulty walking say that their other capabilities or complaints aren't recognized. Rachel Smiley, for instance, who spent forty-five years as a missionary and teacher in South America and another fifteen years after that as a librarian at the Light and Life School in Los Angeles, is still an active reader and thinker. Now, because she can't walk very well, she uses a walker. "When people see me, they take it for granted that I can't see or hear," she says with a wry smile. "They just assume I've deteriorated in other ways as well as in my ability to walk." Rachel, who has excellent hearing and sight, accepts the fact that she can't walk well, but resents being given infirmities she doesn't have.

When physicians have "ageist" attitudes, older patients have reason to question whether they will get proper treatment—and whether, in a life-threatening situation, as much as possible will be done to save their lives.

"I resent the attitude of some doctors that they wouldn't do for me what they would do for someone younger," says Rachel's eighty-two-year-old sister-in-law, Faith Smiley. "They might say, 'Well, she's eighty-two, she doesn't have that much longer to live anyway.' How do they know? I might have another twenty years! Recently I heard someone on television get asked how long she wanted to live. She said, 'I want to live as long as I'm alive!' That's just how I feel. And the longer the better!"

Whether they come from the doctor, the patient, or the patient's family, stereotypes about aging interfere with good health care and good treatment. The health of older people, just like the health of younger people, isn't static. We feel better or worse physically at different times, and we change in other ways, too. Poor health and aging do *not* go hand in hand. Think over what you believe about aging and then question your assumptions. They interfere with clear observation and further complicate treatment. Remember that often your deeply held myths also represent a fear: "This will happen to me when I get old." Even if a certain disease happened to your mother or father, it doesn't mean it will happen to you.

THE MYTH OF SENILITY

The biggest *myth* about aging is that if you live long enough, you'll get senile. According to one Harris poll, 45 percent of the Americans surveyed aspired to live to be one hundred but feared longevity because they were afraid of becoming debilitated and senile.

Many older people report that when they forget something important, they panic. "For a while there, I kept thinking, 'Oh, no! It's here! I'm getting senile,' " said May Weston, an eighty-four-year-old Philadelphian who had just come from a lecture on Alzheimer's disease. "Now I'm beginning to realize that unless it's happening to me all the time, in almost every way, it's not senility. I've always been forgetful, and I still am. I do tend to forget that even when I was young, even when I was twenty, I wasn't always fully attentive!"

The *reality* is that cognitive loss, or loss of brain function, is *not* a normal part of aging. Most people's memory function is unchanged their entire adult life, except when they're tired or strained. (Remember, almost no one, young or old, has total recall!) Sometimes, when there are changes in memory, they're not in any way related to aging. If you're disoriented or forgetting things, or if you're having trouble concentrating, it could be from stress, your medications, the fact that you're depressed, or a number of other factors. If a friend or spouse dies or if you've gone through some other major change in your life, disorientation is to be expected, no matter how old you are. It happens to people of all ages and isn't permanent.

Dementia, popularly referred to as "senility," on the other hand, is a disease. It is a diagnosis applied to people who suffer neurological damage, memory loss, mental confusion as to time and place or spells of dizziness. They show a lack of self-care or an inability to do things like pay bills or remember in which direction to turn or how to carry on an ordinary conversation. *None of these things is an ordinary part of age-related changes.*

Delirium

It's all too common to assume that an older person acting confused and disoriented, forgetful, or unable to carry out ordinary tasks is "getting senile"—and that the condition is untreatable. Without a diagnostic workup and evaluation, many an uninformed doctor has automatically given an older person a diagnosis of dementia, confirming the family's worst fears and resulting in a mental-hospital or nursing-home admission. Unfortunately, in these cases, the diagnosis is often based on observable symptoms that are, in fact, treatable and should be called *pseudodementia* (meaning "resembling dementia"). The underlying causes for pseudodementia, as we've said, can be anxiety, stress, depression, or confusion induced by medications. Malnourishment can also create or compound memory loss, as can certain vitamin deficiencies or thyroid disease.

Hundreds of thousands of older people suffer disorientation, mental loss, or dementia from medications they take to "help" them. Researchers are finding all too often that these problems are caused by sleeping pills, minor tranquilizers, ulcer medications, or drugs prescribed for high blood pressure, chronic anxiety, or gastrointestinal complaints. If the medicine was changed or discontinued, the mental problem would "miraculously" disappear.

Changes in a person's mental status can happen quickly or over a long period of time. The "demented" behavior of an older person may include confusion, hallucinations, and a near total lack of recall. Some doctors estimate that perhaps 50 percent of the acute changes in mental functioning in older people have a remedial, arrestable, or reversible cause. Even those that are chronic and misdiagnosed as dementia often have a treatable underlying cause. Many times these changes have come about slowly and may not be as noticeable to the patient or the people around him. Acute changes are usually noticed immediately. Many times a gallbladder attack; a viral infection; heart, kidney, or liver disease—and even appendicitis—can be the source of acute confusion or disorientation in the older person. When the condition is treated, the confusion clears up. If only the mental/emotional symptoms are treated, however, and if the underlying physiological diseases are not adequately diagnosed and treated, the patient's mental functioning can be permanently damaged.

This is potentially quite dangerous for older people, who are in no condition to speak up for themselves when they're mentally and emotionally confused by an underlying and treatable condition. What's particularly distressing is that the same behavior exhibited by a younger person would be promptly questioned, dealt with, and relieved. It would be clear that any younger person exhibiting such behavior had something seriously wrong, and every avenue would be explored before a determination was made about their disease and treatment. Many times, in the case of older people, an inquiry is never even considered.

Nonreversible Dementia

While many forms of dementia can be treated and reversed, there are also those forms that we all fear, those that aren't reversible. The one most in the news and on our minds is Alzheimer's disease, a neurodegenerative disease that affects those parts of the brain that mediate memory, personality, and speech. Victims of Alzheimer's begin to lose their memories quite early in the course of this disease.

According to the Alzheimer's Association, some four million Americans currently have Alzheimer's disease. While most people will not be victims of Alzheimer's, it does appear there's been a dramatic increase in the number of people in the general population who have it. According to research published in the *Journal of the American Medical Association* in November 1989, approximately 10 percent of people sixty-five and older actually get Alzheimer's. The same study asserts that the incidence of Alzheimer's after the age of eighty-five increases to nearly fifty percent. While diagnostic techniques for Alzheimer's are much improved, there's some speculation that this startling number may be inflated due to drug-induced dementias or incorrect diagnoses.

"The average person can rest reassured that most people will not get this disease," says Dr. Andrew L. Lautin of the New York Institute on Aging. "Some patients are concerned and want to be tested. Even though they've had no memory loss, they seem to need the assurance from a diagnostic workup and evaluation that they're okay." He points out that if you aren't deteriorating, there's no reason to take a test because you don't have the illness.

When someone does have a dreaded neurodegenerative disease associated with dementia—be it Alzheimer's, Parkinson's, or Huntington's disease, or an alcohol-related dementia, which is not that uncommon—the prognosis is grave. (Of course, this does not include drug-induced "diseases," which, in fact, can be "cured" if they have been caused by medication. Too often, doctors fail to suspect medication; instead, they make a new diagnosis and then add a second drug to treat the Parkinson's or dementia caused by the first drug.) True neurodegenerative diseases seem to be all or nothing, and people who have them will continue to deteriorate. Alzheimer's, for instance, is not just forgetting names or incidents; it's an unequivocal, uncontestable, obvious change that family and friends notice—including memory loss, reduced attention span, and loss of orientation as to time, place, and person that gets progressively worse. In fact, it's not the patients who usually initiate the diagnostic workup for neurodegenerative diseases. It's family or friends, who have noticed a severe incapacitation and a decreased ability to interact with others.

Parkinson's disease occurs when an area of the brain called the "substantia nigra" inexplicably stops functioning. Patients become stiff, have difficulty initiating movements, and have tremors in their hands, arms, faces, and legs. In the final phases of Parkinson's disease, patients seem to become frozen in place. About half a million Americans are currently suffering from Parkinson's disease. Some recent research by Dr. William Davis Parker Jr. and his colleagues at the University of Colorado School of Medicine in Denver suggests that the side effects of three drugs commonly used to treat schizophrenia (haloperidol, chlorpromazine, and thiothixene) create long-term neurological complications that strongly resemble Parkinson's disease or tardive dyskinesia, an uncontrollable writhing.

Patients with neurodegenerative diseases such as Alzheimer's, Creutzfeldt-Jakob, or later stages of Lou Gehrig's disease (amyotrophic lateral sclerosis) usually reach a point where they begin to deteriorate rapidly. There is no reversal. Their memory is dramatically affected in all spheres. They lose their ability to conceptualize basic things—including the learned movements involved in walking and eating and going to the bathroom. As some of the neurons drop out, they may also lose control of their emotions, since part of the function of the brain is to inhibit certain areas of itself. As a result, they may act "crazy." So far, no one knows why the neurons of the brain become so disturbed and cease to function. Research may lead to an understanding of the cause, and thus the solution, but as yet, there's no specific treatment that medicine can offer as a cure to these diseases. Medicine is used mostly to alleviate some of the uncontrolled "crazy behavior" that has been caused by the lack of brain function. These medications are often derived from antipsychotic drugs used for younger people.

AN ABUNDANCE OF MYTHS ON AGING

Although other myths and fears about aging lag far behind the fear of senility, they still interfere with older people feeling good about themselves and getting the quality of health care that they deserve. Some of the most common myths inhibit self-confidence. In fact, by equating images of decrepitude and weakness with advancing years, they invoke feelings of shame about being old. Fear of becoming incapacitated or inept also dampens enthusiasm for learning new skills, undertaking challenging intellectual tasks, and pursuing new adventures. Here's a look at some ideas that inhibit our pride in growing older:

MYTH: Old people lose their memories and their minds. They have great difficulty learning new ideas and are incapable of mastering new concepts. They shouldn't work because basically they've used up their brain power and their capacity to be creative or productive.
REALITY: Aging does *not* produce mental deterioration. In fact, tests of general information and vocabulary frequently show increased capacity with age. Some researchers have likened the mind and memory to muscles that simply need to be exercised to stay in shape. The more they're exercised, the more resilient

they are. Those researchers say that years of schooling are better predictors of differences in memory than age is. When there is mental decline or a lack of productivity in an older person, it is usually a result of poor health, boredom, or a lack of motivation. We only have to look at Georgia O'Keefe, Vladimir Horowitz, Oliver Wendell Holmes, and Martha Graham to see that age doesn't limit one's capacity to be vital, creative, and productive.

MYTH: Old people don't have sex. After a certain age, they lose their desire for touching, kissing, and physical pleasure. It's a good thing they're not interested because even if they were, they couldn't do anything about it anyway.
REALITY: Men and women are capable of sexual arousal and orgasm well into their nineties and older. While it may take slightly more time for a man to achieve a full erection or for a woman to lubricate, most older people with partners report that they enjoy sex and have satisfying sexual experiences. Older people want intimacy and close sexual contact as consistently as they ever did, and sometimes even more. No one loses their need for physical love or pleasure because of aging. If you are normally interested in sex and you suddenly lose interest or an ability to perform, it's because of illness, stress, anxiety, depression, medication, or perhaps because you're drinking too much alcohol. Quite a few factors that have nothing to do with aging can affect your sex drive.

MYTH: People lose their physical vigor when they get old. Old people are always weak and tired and short of breath. They have to get used to staying home. They shouldn't expect to enjoy going out as much as they used to because it will just wear them out.
REALITY: Loss of physical vigor is not a normal part of aging. Unless disease prevents it, older people can

be physically energetic all of their lives. Although many older people do experience a slowing down of their heart, lung, and muscle capacity, it doesn't keep them from physical activity. In fact, getting out is stimulating both physically and intellectually. Breathlessness, fainting, or fatigue are not a normal part of aging. Doctors tell us that some ninety-year-olds have cardiovascular systems that show no decline whatsoever. "The notion that the aging cardiovascular system necessarily suffers a big decrease in functional ability just isn't true," says Dr. Edward Lakatta, chief of the Laboratory of Cardiovascular Science at the Gerontology Research Center in Baltimore. "If these symptoms are related to cardiovascular function, they're suggestive of the presence of cardiovascular disease or decondition—not aging per se."

MYTH: As you get older, you need more sleep.
REALITY: In reality, as you get older, you need *less* sleep. It's perfectly normal for sleeping patterns to change with age. Many physicians prescribe sleeping tablets to patients who complain of difficulty sleeping, but nine out of ten times, these prescriptions are incorrect, according to Dr. Charles Herrera, director of the Sleep Disorders Program for the Middle Aged and Older Adults in the Department of Geriatrics at Mount Sinai Medical Center. Most sleep disorders can be treated without drugs. Families of older people should realize that nothing is wrong if they hear their elders getting up in the middle of the night to fix a snack or read a book. Wakefulness, light sleeping, and altered sleep patterns are not a sign of an older person's senility or health problems. They're just signs of adaptation to a normal change of patterns. If you're awake in the night, it's better to get up and enjoy your time than to lie in bed thinking you have to sleep because it's nighttime or worry that you won't be getting enough sleep.

MYTH: Older people regress into childlike states. It's normal for them to be confused and disoriented.

REALITY: It's not normal to be confused, disoriented, or regressed because of age. Sometimes a high temperature in an older person may cause confusion or disorientation that goes away with the normalizing of the temperature. All too often, confusion or disorientation can be traced to medications. If an older person is unable to do things for himself, then something is wrong, and he should be seen by a health-care professional who understands geriatric issues.

MYTH: The longer you live, the sicker you'll get. If you're really old, what do you expect? Just be grateful that you're alive!

REALITY: It's true that your susceptibility to some diseases increases as you age; however, many people in their late eighties or nineties enjoy excellent health. If you eat properly, exercise, have a social network and a sense of self-worth, you will increase your odds, which are already good, of remaining mentally and physically vigorous. Aging associated with sickness is the *pathology* of aging, not normal aging.

MYTH: Older people should expect to be depressed—it comes with the territory.

REALITY: Aging is not the cause of depression. If you haven't been depressed all your life, you don't have to start now. Older people don't have to put up with being depressed or assume that a depression will be permanent.

Social workers Shirley Wickman and Elaine Johannes, case workers for the Area Agency on Aging, which services seventeen rural counties in Kansas, say that doctors, social workers, and the family often attribute depression to aging. "But if you ask the important questions," says Shirley Wickman, "you'll find out what it is. It's usually medications the person is taking that make them sluggish and lethargic, or it's foods or certain life events.'' These are all problems that can be dealt with effectively.

If you are depressed, it may manifest itself in sleep disturbances, early-morning wakenings, crying spells, a decrease in appetite, loss of libido, sad spells, trouble with concentrating, memory loss, or loss of interest in usual pleasures. Talk to your doctor about its possible link to medications or an undiagnosed medical condition. If you are mourning the death of a spouse or a child, the loss of your role in relationship to other people, the loss of your home, or any life event that changes your perception of yourself in the world, remember that depression is a natural reaction. Treatment or counseling can often help. Some doctors estimate, however, that most depressions lift within six to nine months no matter how they're diagnosed or treated.

MYTH: Sooner or later, old people will get constipated and be unable to control their bladders. If they have diarrhea or suddenly lose urine, incontinence is finally catching up with them.
REALITY: These conditions are not a normal part of getting old. If you are constipated, you may not be eating enough roughage, you may have polyps or an obstruction blocking the food, or you may simply need to eat more fruits and vegetables and drink more water. Problems of incontinence can also be solved. Stress, illness, or medicines may be a factor.

MYTH: Old people have to expect to be stiff and have aching bones. They shouldn't take long walks or runs.
REALITY: Skeletal and muscular changes can cause a stiff feeling or pains in the knees and joints. More often than not, however, older people create stiffness for themselves by limiting their activity. You should maximize your activity, physical flexibility, and range of motion through walks and regular exercise.

MYTH: Problems with balance and gait are a normal part of aging.

REALITY: These problems are *not* a normal part of aging. More often than not, they're symptoms of underlying physical, emotional, or environmental situations. Sometimes the problem is as simple as the need for a new prescription for eyeglasses. Other times, the issue is more complex. Balance can be affected by a stroke or a brain tumor. Heart-rhythm disturbances or muscle degeneration can contribute to falling episodes, and neurological diseases such as Parkinson's or Alzheimer's can affect gait and postural stability. All of these conditions can be aggravated by the fear of falling, which can lead to increased social isolation, dependence, and immobility. If you have trouble keeping your balance, talk to your doctor about it.

MYTH: Old people can't expect to hear or see as well as they used to. They might as well get used to the isolation.

REALITY: Visual and hearing impairments are common among people over sixty-five. Studies show that the proportion of the population with twenty-twenty vision diminishes 75 percent between the ages of sixty and eighty, while the proportion whose vision is twenty-fifty or worse more than triples during the same period. A major cause of the visual problems is reduced elasticity of the lens, which makes it difficult to see objects close at hand. Other changes in the eye reduce the amount of light that reaches the retina, which decreases the sharpness of visual images.

Many older people also lose some of their ability to hear higher ranges of sound, which sometimes makes it difficult to perceive nuances of speech.

If you are affected by vision or hearing loss, you don't need to experience isolation because of it. You may need a brighter light for reading, or a prescription for glasses or contact lenses. If visual problems continue or intensify, you may require cataract surgery or other corrective surgery or eye care. Eye surgery today usually involves efficient and effective laser procedures that do not require hospitalization or a long recovery. Most hearing difficulties can be corrected with a hearing aid. In your own home, at least, you can also decrease competing noise that makes it harder to focus on what is being said.

MYTH: Old people like to be alone. They don't like all the hyperactivity of younger people and children.

REALITY: No matter what age we are, we're social creatures. We need to touch and be touched, we need to exchange feelings and ideas with other people. Older people need social contact and need to feel themselves part of a larger community. When older people stop socializing or interacting with their families and friends, it's often symptomatic of hearing or vision loss, immobility, or other illnesses that make them feel they can't venture forth. Sometimes they're sick and are embarrassed about their appearance. Someone who begins to isolate himself or herself is usually displaying a symptom that should be investigated. More often than not, someone who wants to be alone all the time is sick or depressed, and needs contact. This can often be dealt with by getting medical treatment or developing new interests, getting out of the house, joining a social center, taking a course or an exercise class, and establishing or renewing friendships. Certainly, a satisfying social life is an indicator of good health. Studies indicate that people who have active relationships and feel loved live the longest.

WHEN SHOULD YOU SEE THE DOCTOR?

It may be all well and good to run to the doctor with serious symptoms, you may say, but there *are* trivial symptoms that should be ignored. You may wonder exactly how you can determine whether something you're feeling is really a symptom of an illness or just a minor pain that's a normal part of living, such as the bruise you got on your leg from running into the corner of the coffee table or the headache you had the morning after you drank three glasses of red wine.

If you're trying to decide whether or not you should see the doctor, evaluate your condition by reviewing your body and your day-to-day experiences. If you feel something is not right, try to identify exactly what isn't right about what you're feeling. Ask yourself the following questions:

- Is this problem compromising the way I live?
- Is it making me more tired?
- Is it affecting my life-style?
- Is it affecting my activities?
- Am I having problems eating?
- Am I having problems walking? dressing myself?
- Am I having problems talking?
- Is it affecting my vision? my memory? the way I go to the bathroom?
- Is it affecting my attitude? my personality?
- Is there any particular time of day that the problem is most noticeable?

"We tell people to go to the doctor if they experience any of the four *M*'s," says Dr. Douglas Young, former medical director of Geriatrics at HCA Wesley Medical Center in Wichita, Kansas. "The *M*'s are: *mind*—any change in your mental status; *meals*—any change in your ability to eat; *mobility*—any change in your balance or ability to move around; or *micturition*—any change in your urination. Any of those four are direct indications that something is wrong. This is particularly true for the frail elderly.''

If you are having a pain, be prepared to answer questions about the way the pain feels: Is it a dull pain? a sharp pain? Does it go away quickly? Do certain situations make it go away or come back? Does it radiate to any other area; for example, does the pain in your chest travel to your arm? Is there any particular time of day that you notice the pain?

As you age, you'll notice normal changes that take place in your body. Some of these changes will be directly related to aging, while others are related to illness. Rather than making a major and potentially life-threatening decision yourself, as Dominick Lepore did when he waited months to call the doctor about the pain in his chest and his episodes of passing out, it's wise to let the doctor make that decision for you. If the discomfort is a result of a normal process of aging, the doctor can suggest ways to accommodate your life or make adjustments or changes for optimal functioning. If, on the other hand, you have an illness, then you have the advantage of having reported it early. It can be dealt with, and you'll know how to plan for it.

''If you think any particular symptom or persistent problem is due to your age, go to the doctor,'' says Dr. Young in Wichita. ''Otherwise you may let the problem go on so long that it's too late for something to be done about it.''

If your doctor says you should expect to feel the way you do (no matter how much pain you're in) because you're over sixty-five, seventy-five, eighty-five, or ninety-five, you may have to set him straight or find another doctor. If, however, thorough medical workups reveal that you have a condition or discomfort you are going to have to live with at your age, there are both positive and negative ways of dealing with your situation.

"If the doctor says, 'These are your limitations,' you may hear it as all negative—'You can't do this,' or 'You have to give up that,' " says gerontologist Sylvia McBurnie, who's an assistant professor of Nursing at SUNY, The Health Science Center at Brooklyn's College of Nursing. "But there are ways to look at limitations in a positive light. You can still enjoy your life; there are simply adjustments you have to make to have more comfort, more safety. For instance, you may need to remove slippery rugs so that you don't fall. If your eyesight is poorer than it used to be, you will need brighter lights for reading and perhaps more powerful reading glasses. If you walk more slowly, you may need to plan to give yourself more time going and coming to social events and appointments."

If you encounter a doctor who has hackneyed views on what you're experiencing or takes lightly what you're saying—or if you feel he doesn't understand your concerns and priorities—tell him that you know there are certain things that will change as you age, but that you also know there's no reason for you to experience pain or discomfort.

Ask the doctor, "Are there any kinds of tests you feel are necessary to discover whether my symptoms are due to normal aging or because of illness?" or tell him, "I know how I usually feel, and this is very different." Blood tests, EKGs, X rays, CAT scans, and many other diagnostic tools at the doctor's disposal can objectively measure your condition.

If you're not satisfied with the doctor's response, you don't have to accept it. You're entitled to a second opinion or a different doctor.

Don't Compromise Your Own Interests
Remember that for the most part, it's *not* normal to feel pain or to feel extremely weak. It's *not* normal to black out or to have time periods you can't account for! It's

not normal to feel sick to your stomach most of the time or to pass blood in your stools.

You may be afraid of what you'll find out if you see the doctor, but it probably won't be as bad as you imagined. If your condition can be treated, you will soon feel better and more like yourself again. If you have a problem that can't be treated, you can learn how to adjust your life-style. Taking action will put you in command again.

Often, the doctor will be able to tell you what caused your problem and how it can be dealt with effectively. Preventive measures might involve improving your nutritional state, exercising more, resting more, using a cane, not sleeping so much, taking your medicine correctly, or reporting the symptoms earlier. If you've had a problem, ask the doctor, ''What kinds of things can I do to prevent this from happening again?''

No matter how old you are, it's important to see a health-care professional when you don't feel well or when an uncomfortable or painful condition doesn't go away. Don't ever refuse to see a doctor because you imagine what you're feeling is ''just a symptom of old age.'' Don't take anything for granted or assume that you have to compromise your interests or your good health just because you're getting older.

CHAPTER 3

Rx: Prescriptions for Your Health

> "Doctors pour drugs of which they know little, to cure diseases of which they know less, into human beings of whom they know nothing."
>
> —VOLTAIRE

Unfortunately, there's still a great deal of truth to Voltaire's observation, especially for the older population, who consume a third of more than 1.7 billion prescriptions dispensed in the United States annually. At an estimated twenty doses in each prescription, that means that people sixty-five and older in this country are swallowing a minimum of ten billion prescribed doses a year.

"It's a simple fact that older people are on too many medicines," says Dr. John W. Rowe, president of the Mount Sinai Medical Center. "What I don't like is that the currency of the relationship between the physician and the older person has become the prescription pad."

Dr. James Cooper at the College of Pharmacy at the University of Georgia agrees. "When a doc says, 'Let's try these three medicines and see what happens,' it's like saying, 'We'll fix the cut when it happens,' instead of 'Let's remove the razor before it cuts the skin,' " he says. "Many times, these medication problems occur with older people because their physicians are geared toward 'crisis care'—let a crisis happen and then deal with it—instead of toward preventive medicine and long-term treatment."

The power to "cure" is a powerful incentive to prescribe. "Doctors are accustomed to treating younger patients with acute problems,'' says Dr. Cooper. ''One way of handling those problems is to give them drugs, 'cure' them, and get them back on their feet. Physicians haven't traditionally been trained in ways of managing ongoing problems, such as arthritis or heart problems that cannot be 'cured' but must be adapted to in ways least debilitating to one's life-style.''

THE POWER OF THE CURE

The number of prescriptions being given to older people may also reflect a change in medical philosophy from a passive to a more active role, a change that is the result of recent strides in medical therapeutics. Doctors are responding in many ways to their newfound power to define and effectively treat diseases. Now, for instance, a physician can prescribe medications to *prevent* heart attacks and strokes.

Quite recently, physicians have also gained the power to reduce mortality and morbidity from heart attacks, because of thrombolytic therapy. It is now known that ninety percent of heart attacks are caused by a clot that forms around a coronary artery where a piece of plaque has ruptured. So, when a heart attack occurs and a victim seeks immediate treatment, a physician can inject the patient with a thrombolytic drug—a ''clot buster'' that dissolves the clot and prevents further clotting and tissue damage. This ''clot buster'' saves lives.

''It used to be that the medicines never worked very well and side effects were worse than any benefits,'' says internist Dr. Barbara Otto. ''But now more prescriptions can be given because diseases are more specifically defined, and appropriate therapy for them has been established.

''Hypertension is a good example. Physicians knew all along that it was important to treat hypertension, but they didn't know when to start or how vigorous to be, and they didn't have the drugs to do it. Now they know that hypertension should be treated; it's defined as a systolic blood pressure [on the top end] that is greater than 140 millimeters of mercury [Hg] and the diastolic blood pressure [the resting blood pressure] as greater than 90mm of mercury [Hg]. We didn't know that before! We also know now that morbidity and mortality can be changed by treating the high blood pressure, and we know that you should try to control it. Now we have dozens of drugs to treat hypertension. That's gratifying, and it accounts for a significant increase in the number of prescriptions currently being written.''

The large number of available drugs also influences the increased number of prescriptions being consumed by older people, since the physician can choose from a vast number that allow him to treat a particular condition. It used to be that if patients needed but couldn't tolerate Inderal, for instance, there was no other beta-blocker (a drug that blocks the heart's response to adrenalin and reduces high blood pressure) for them to take. Now there are at least a dozen beta-blockers with slightly different effects; a physician can go from one to the next until he finds out which one works best for that particular patient.

Another factor in the increase in medications being used may stem directly from the scale of advertising and marketing being conducted by the pharmaceutical industry. Pharmaceutical companies advertise their products directly to the doctor—and are an important source of drug information. According to Morton Mintz in *The Therapeutic Nightmare*, the pharmaceutical industry spends one dollar out of one hundred for research, while spending seven dollars on advertising to doctors.

THE PRESCRIPTION AS A LOLLIPOP

Probably one of the single most significant reasons for overmedication comes from the fact that the prescription is commonly used for "closure" of a patient's visit with the doctor. When the doctor puts his pen on the prescription pad and begins to write, it's the traditional signal for both the doctor and the patient that the medical visit is ending. For the doctor, who might have difficulty communicating well, it's a painless way of moving the patient out of the office and making room for the next person on the schedule. For the patient, the prescription becomes the physical representation of his visit to the doctor. It's the reward, the symbolic "lollipop" that the patient gets to take with him when he leaves.

Some patients aren't satisfied with less than that "lollipop" because they believe that the answer to whatever ails them can be found in a bottle of pills. While the doctor might be doing them a favor *not* to give them a prescription every time, many people feel as if they have been cheated or that the doctor hasn't earned his pay if he doesn't write a prescription.

"People are disappointed if the doctor doesn't give them medicine," says Dr. Rowe. "If they come away from an office visit without a prescription, they think the doctor's not using his expertise. When they go to the doctor with complaints that they're not sleeping properly, for instance, they don't want to hear that it's normal for their sleeping habits to change.

"The best advice I could give older people is don't expect and require that your physician give you medicine for every problem," says Dr. Rowe. "Expect a diagnosis before you get a treatment."

The trouble with the number of prescriptions older people use is financial as well as medical. While all their health-care expenses are higher as a result of the negative side effects of using too many medications, their drug expenditures alone are particularly pronounced.

"It's not unusual for an older person to have two thousand to three thousand dollars in drug costs in one year," says Dr. William Campbell at the University of Washington's School of Pharmacy Practice in Seattle. "It's a tremendous financial issue for them—particularly since most of them are on limited budgets, and Medicare doesn't pay for outpatient prescriptions. Also, because of inappropriate use, misinformation, and poor prescribing, they're particularly vulnerable to the adverse effects of drugs. It's a tough problem."

An Alternative Approach

Although I heard many complaints about doctors giving prescriptions over the phone, about "weekend doctors" doubling medications without knowing what else the patient was taking, and doctors prescribing three or more drugs that have known adverse interactions, I also heard stories about doctors who never fell into the trap of using the prescription pad as a substitute for careful diagnosis and patient communication.

Consulting pharmacist Randall Wright of Kansas City told me a story about a physician he once worked with named Dr. Clinton B. Hash, who educated his patients to use medicine sparingly and with supervision.

Dr. Hash, who practiced in Seneca, Kansas, for more than thirty years, used to give people "little yellow football pills" if they had headaches, pulled shoulders, arthritis, or a backache. After diagnosing minor muscular, skeletal, or arthritic pains, Dr. Hash gave prescriptions according to the following formula: If you were the man of the family—a big man who was a farmer or former football player—you took one yellow football pill. If you were the grown woman in the family, you took one-half of a football pill. If you were the child, you got one-fourth to one-half of the football pill.

Babies could have a little shaving scraped off after a call to the doctor.

Dr. Hash never prescribed more than ten to twenty pills to one family at a time. "He said, 'If you give people a lot of pills, they'll take a lot of pills,' " Randall Wright recalls. " 'If you don't want people to take a lot of pills, you won't give them a lot of pills.'

"Dr. Hash and I had made a tacit agreement that we wouldn't tell people what was in the yellow football pill," he said. "Dr. Hash had set up in people's minds that this was an extremely strong medicine—so strong that a big man could have only one and his wife could only have one-half. But what was actually in this yellow football pill was everyday, run-of-the-mill five grains of aspirin.

"Dr. Hash had been giving them out at an extremely low dosage to treat all kinds of aches and pains and even arthritis. He was able to teach people by example that medicines were something to be handled with great caution. It turned out that shortly after Dr. Hash died, the yellow football pills stopped being produced. They were replaced in Seneca by white basketball pills—which actually were aspirin tablets. But people in Seneca still had to go to the doctor to get a prescription for them."

Although Dr. Hash's paternalistic methods might be questionable, his conservative approach is appropriate. Today, too many doctors are tempted to be too liberal in the numbers and dosages of medications they prescribe. They choose among thousands of different kinds of little yellow football pills, white basketball pills, red kidney-shaped pills, blue oblong pills, blue round pills, and an assortment of other colors and shapes and liquids and suppositories and topical medications. The choice is tempting because of their potential effectiveness and because sometimes they provide quick answers to difficult questions. Pharmaceutical companies are constantly at work developing new and better formulas and marketing them to physicians. Physicians are prescribing them to their patients, and patients are buying them from pharmacies and taking them home.

WHAT IS A PRESCRIPTION?

"Prescription" merely defines the legal status of a drug. Under the medical system we've established during this century, a prescription drug must be ordered by a licensed physician—a medical doctor, osteopath, or dentist. Pharmacists, chiropractors, midwives, housewives, or nurses cannot prescribe medications as they once did. Sometimes physicians prescribe a "nonprescription" drug as well. In other words, they order an over-the-counter drug such as aspirin, which can be bought without a prescription. When your doctor prescribes an over-the-counter drug, it's usually because he thinks it will be useful and he wants you to take the medication under his supervision.

Certainly, for thousands of years before there were any legal strictures about the administration of drugs, there were medicines to treat illnesses. An early Egyptian medical reference book, the *Ebers Papyrus*, lists some nine hundred prescriptions that were used in the time of the Pharaoh Amenhotep (about 1600 B.C.). As far back as we've studied the habits of man, we've been able to see that tribal healers, shamans, and physicians have used different substances—many reputed to have magical powers—to make people feel better when they were feverish or in pain, anxious, melancholy, or "losing their strength." Women in childbirth were given certain potions to drink. The sap from various barks was put on wounds. Healers foraged for plants, roots, herbs, barks, chalks, and berries that could be mixed, boiled, scraped, or chewed to help cure specific conditions. Many of those substances form the basis for medications that doctors still use to heal and restore the

body. Digitalis, for instance, used to be squeezed from
the foxglove plant. American Indians alleviated pain by
chewing willow bark, which has the same active ingredient, salicylate, that we find in aspirin. Even though
some of the substances are still natural, most medicines
we use today are synthetics. As Dr. James Long, author
of *The Essential Guide to Prescription Drugs*, points
out, these chemicals are useful in treatment ''because
a particular aspect of their chemical interactions within
the body favorably modifies some tissue structure or
function. This, in turn, assists natural mechanisms that
heal and restore. Drug actions alone do not 'cure' disease. They benefit the patient by making a significant
contribution to the total scheme of processes needed to
restore health.''

How Does Medicine Work?
Okay, you might ask, but just how does medicine really
work in the body? Just what is medicine and what does
it do?

When I started trying to think about the whole process of drugs and the body, I felt like a city kid who
couldn't visualize that the white liquid she poured into
her glass from a carton originally came from a cow. I
decided to go see some medicines made, so I went to
visit Squibb, a large pharmaceutical manufacturer based
in New Jersey. This company was started in 1858 by an
apothecary and physician named Edward Robinson
Squibb, who invented a process of distilling ether by
steam, making the use of anesthesia during surgery possible and reliable.

At the Squibb research laboratories and manufacturing plant in New Brunswick, New Jersey, I donned a
plastic hat to cover my hair, and walked with other
white-capped people through wide, sterile stainless-steel
halls and rooms. I watched hypertension pills being
made through large glass windows that reminded me of
nursery windows in hospitals, where you look in to see

the newborn babies. In those sterile rooms, I saw enormous machines that looked like huge silver malted-milk containers or small space capsules. They rotated around and around as hundreds of thousands of gallons of chemicals were measured into them by meticulous computer controls and then blended, spun, and mixed. Inside the containers, liquids and powders were being transformed into granules that were transformed again, one stage after another, into millions and millions of small white pills. These pills were then dumped into large carts and wheeled into even larger rooms, where they were thrown into machines that looked like gigantic dryers. A colored liquid was fed into those machines, so that, as literally millions of white pills swirled and swayed around and around in the dryers, they were coated in blue color. Eventually they were such a bright, shiny, dry blue they looked as if they'd been born blue and were blue through to the core.

A Medicine's Journey

Afterward I tried to imagine the route the blue hypertension pill would travel as it made its way into a person's system. I could see the blue pill move into the pink-white cavern of the patient's mouth and travel down her throat. If we could look at a cross-section of her body, we would see beautiful colors—all the tissues and arteries and veins and an assortment of chemicals that have been organized into the very effective systems that make up human beings. The blue pill travels down through the narrow esophagus to the stomach, where it's dissolved by stomach acids. Then the particles travel into the small bowel, where they're absorbed into the bloodstream and distributed to their sites of action, where they perform their jobs. Most medicines are then excreted by the kidney or metabolized (changed and broken down) by the liver and then excreted by the kidney. From the liver, what remains of the dissolved drug flows into the receiving chamber of the heart and then is eventually pumped back out through the bloodstream to all the tissues of the body.

A Medicine's Function

The idea of using drugs from outside to alter the course of an interior illness intrigued me. Once I could imagine how it *looked* to swallow a pill and what course the medicine took through the body, I tried to imagine how the medicine actually *worked* to make a difference within the system. Dr. Donald L. Nathanson in Philadelphia and Dr. Barbara Otto in New York each helped me reach an understanding of the process.

To begin to think about the function of medicine within the body, let's think about the whole system. From this particular perspective, the body is basically a large bag of chemicals. Some of the chemicals are organized into walls and compartments (tissues and organs) that hold them in separate places. Everything within the body is an atom or molecule.

Looking at the way chemicals work in our bodies, let's figure out what we need to function normally and to keep the chemicals balanced properly. Let's look, for instance, at iodine. We human beings need iodine for the thyroid gland to operate normally. Traditionally, it was supplied by the diet when most people lived near the ocean. When we became industrialized and had transportation, however, people moved away from the sea to inland areas such as the Midwest, where there isn't any fresh seafood or seaweed. As they moved away from the ocean, their intake of iodine decreased, and they became iodine-deficient. It was only then that the problem of one of the glands of the body—the thyroid gland, which is dependent upon iodine—became manifest. People in the Midwest, and in countries like Switzerland, got goiters because their thyroids didn't have enough iodine. The goiter would grow very large in an attempt to get the iodine the gland needed. It's for that reason that we have iodized salt. It adds a chemical, iodine, to offset what we're not getting in our diet.

A Delicate Balance

Sometimes we need to take certain chemicals out of our bodies to stay healthy. Other times we need to add them.

Depending on the disease, we add or subtract chemicals to keep the balance. Some chemicals replace essential nutrients. Some try to correct metabolic errors. For example, if the thyroid gland in the base of the neck is not producing enough thyroxine to properly regulate the body's metabolism, thyroid hormone (thyroxine), estrogen, and testosterone are often used as hormone replacement therapies. On the other hand, if the thyroid is secreting too much thyroxine, drugs are used to reduce the thyroxine and return hormone levels to normal.

Other times, when the body fails to remove uric acid from the bloodstream, a drug is given to cause the kidney to flush it out, while another drug can be given to stop the uric acid from forming. A doctor may prescribe allopurinol to prevent the formation of excess uric acid and probenecid to eliminate excess uric acid. Or doctors may prescribe cimetidine (Tagamet) to prevent excess acid, while antacids such as Maalox or Mylanta are used to neutralize excess stomach acid once it is formed.

Some medicines give the body a chance to correct itself, while others maintain balance in an otherwise unstable system. Anti-inflammatory drugs such as ibuprofen, aspirin, and naproxen, for instance, basically work to stop the redness and swelling that are caused by the body's reaction to injury or irritation. Anti-inflammatory drugs have also been found to counteract prostaglandins, which produce pain. Thus, they are taken to relieve symptoms such as inflammation, swelling, stiffness, and joint pain caused by arthritis or rheumatism. They also are used to relieve other kinds of pain or to treat painful conditions such as bursitis, tendonitis, or sprains and strains.

Some antihypertensive drugs work by relaxing the walls of the small arteries, known as arterioles, while others remove salt and water to reduce the blood volume that causes the pressure. Antidepressants may alter the balance of the brain chemicals that normally make us feel good and that change when we are depressed.

We put other chemicals, such as antibiotics, into the body to fight off certain diseases or bacteria. When you have an infection, for instance, it means that certain bacteria have gotten past your body's defense system. If you take penicillin, it interferes with the formation of the cell wall and prevents the bacteria from multiplying. Human cells do not have cell walls, so the drug is harmless in human cells. When a person has cancer, some of his cells change from their normal state into alien cells that multiply rapidly, out of control. Chemotherapy kills those cancer cells that are rapidly multiplying. Since cancer cells are similar to normal human cells, the cancer drugs also can kill other rapidly multiplying cells indiscriminately—which is why chemotherapy causes so many things, such as hair loss, to happen to the body.

I now understand that when a physician gives a particular chemical to try to improve a patient's condition, we call it a drug. Every medicine that is given is part of an involved process trying to affect a particular biological system. Basically, the way medicine works in the human body involves complex relationships between substances balanced in a very sophisticated system.

DRUGS DON'T ALWAYS HIT THE BULLSEYE

When medicines are advisable, the "drug of choice" is the one that, in the judgment of the doctor, is most likely to produce positive effects. "This selection—the best drug, in the right dose, for the right person, at the right time—is the crucial first step in the successful use of drugs," says Dr. James Long in *The Essential Guide to Prescription Drugs*. "But this decision can never be made with complete assurance that the interactions of drug, patient, and disease will be exactly as intended or predicted. When a patient takes any prescribed drug for the first time, he or she is in fact participating in an experiment under the physician's direction. While the physician's knowledge of the patient's general condition, his or her current illness, and the actions of the drug make it possible to predict the probable (and certainly the desirable) course of the experiment, the full consequences can never be foreseen. There's always an inescapable element of uncertainty."

Pharmaceutical companies may spend millions of dollars and many years on the development of each new drug, but exactly how that drug will work within the individual's body is still unknown. This is true despite the stringent precautions that have come from the drug having been subjected to hundreds of hours of tests, quality control, and measures by the FDA to prove its safety and effectiveness. Until a drug has been on the market many years, not much is known about its long-term effects, particularly when it comes to the response that drug will create within the older person's unpredictable body. If it's a drug meant to affect the gastric system, will the way it metabolizes also have an effect on the pumping of the heart?

When I talked to Dr. Berhard Mehl at Mount Sinai Hospital about "drug targets" and how different systems "compete" for the drug-receptor site, I realized that a drug can be similar to a drunk and inexperienced marksman aiming his shotgun at one particular target in the middle of a busy intersection. The marksman (the drug) aims at the target (the heart, for example) but lets off a volley that hits many other unintended targets as well. The bullets are delivered by the bloodstream everywhere in the body. Molecules aimed for the heart may make the victim sleepy when they hit the brain, while the effect on the liver may be quite another matter. An antihypertensive medicine can also hit mood controls and cause the patient to feel depressed. Dr. Mehl pointed out that drugs are now being targeted more specifically, and more successfully, than they used to be. Tagamet, for instance, is very effective in going straight to work on ulcers. But even Tagamet can scatter into unwanted territory. One of its major side effects is mental confusion, especially in older people, who may eliminate the drug more slowly. A good example of a drug that doesn't scatter is radioactive iodine, which is given to treat cancer of the thyroid. High doses are harder to eliminate and may create even greater problems. Because the thyroid gland soaks up iodine so rapidly, it isn't dispersed to other parts of the body. Even with the progress that's been made, however, the pharmaceutical industry still has a lot of target practice ahead of it before it's certain of consistently hitting the mark.

Sometime after I understood this image of the way drugs are targeted, a physician friend told me that in the medical world, doctors often refer to "the magic bullet"—a term for any medication that one hopes will magically hit the mark. "You just close your eyes and pray," she said, "because you never really know."

Another friend of mine, who had witnessed his wife's critical but ultimately successful bout with leukemia, said that he had thought of her chemotherapy as a good guy with a machine gun who was chasing an evil thief. The evil thief disappeared into a large crowd standing on a corner at Times Square. The good guy gunned down hundreds of perfectly innocent people in his hopes that he would kill the evil thief in the process.

"Even with the best intentions in the world," says Mr. Hugo Koch at the National Center for Health Statistics, "doctors can't know the full consequences of the multiple use of drugs—even the Food and Drug Administration doesn't know it." On some level, he agreed, when it comes to drug use, we're all guinea pigs.

Unfortunately, too many older people find that their participation in what could be called the great drug-prescribing experiments of the 1980s is difficult, distressing, and sometimes deadly. Even if medicines help the vast majority, says Dr. Peter Lamy at the University of Maryland at Baltimore, the people who are adversely affected are far too numerous. Even if fatal adverse reactions were relatively uncommon, an adverse reaction is unacceptable to the person who experiences it.

There is no diabolical plan here. Doctors don't intentionally overmedicate or give prescriptions that harm instead of help. In fact, there's evidence that most doctors try very hard to be careful. In their study of 135 million prescriptions written by doctors to patients sixty-five and over who had come into their offices for visits in 1980 to 1981, the National Center for Health Statistics found in its National Ambulatory Medical Care Survey that, contrary to popular myth, physicians generally were very cautious in determining and following up on prescriptions. Although they did prescribe an average of 1.64 drugs per visit for their older patients (compared to the 0.9 prescriptions they wrote for their patients under seventy-five), they gave specific follow-up instructions and scheduled return visits to evaluate dosages and reactions to the medication. They monitored and adjusted dosages and changed medications if necessary.

In spite of their efforts, however, the main complaint that brought patients to the doctor's office was *dizziness*—which, as we mentioned before, is one of the most frequent major signals of an adverse drug reaction. Also high on the list of complaints presented by aging patients were "blurred vision" (listed second) and "general weakness" (listed eighth).

"There was little pathological basis for the dizziness, for many of the vision problems, and for much of the general weakness," said Mr. Hugo Koch of the National Center for Health Statistics, who evaluated the drug data from this vast and comprehensive study. "In part, these symptoms probably were caused or aggravated by the body's reaction to drugs—especially to their multiple use."

Mr. Koch conceded that the average of 1.6 drugs per visit found by his study probably understated the actual extent to which multiple medication occurred among these older office patients. For example, the survey did not account for telephone refills, which are sometimes used in the management of certain chronic diseases, or for unreported self-medication with over-the-counter drugs such as analgesics, anti-inflammatory agents, antacids, and laxatives. He said that the older office patient might be taking an average of at least two to three drugs at one time, if not more. One of the known truths of our times is that *the more medications you take, the more likely you are to have adverse reactions to them*.

THE PRESCRIPTIONS THEMSELVES

Many of the 567 million or more prescriptions older Americans fill every year are for "fine tuning" comfort levels, while others are directly involved in treating acute illnesses or managing chronic conditions. They can be correlated with the most common diagnoses for older people who are living at home and seeing the doctor at his or her office.

In their study of eighty-two million office visits made in 1980 and 1981 by people seventy-five and older who lived in the community, the National Ambulatory Medical Care Survey found that circulatory problems were by far the most common. As the main diagnosis recorded by the doctor or as a secondary problem coexisting with another main diagnosis, circulatory disease was present at 55 percent of the visits, a fact that becomes dramatically evident when we look at the following list of the ten specific diagnoses most frequently associated with these office visits:

1. Essential hypertension
2. Chronic ischemic heart disease (a narrowing or constriction of the blood vessels that causes a fall in blood supply to the heart muscle and a lack of oxygen to the heart)
3. Diabetes mellitus
4. Osteoarthritis and allied disorders
5. Cataracts
6. Heart failure (can be due to 2, 7 or 10)
7. Cardiac arrhythmia (irregular heartbeat)
8. Arthropathy (arthritis and other related diseases)
9. Glaucoma
10. Hypertensive heart disease (an effect on the heart caused by chronic hypertension).

The ten most frequently prescribed drugs given in those same years were related directly to the ten most frequent diagnoses.

In looking at the ten most frequently prescribed drugs filled in 1991 by the AARP Pharmacy Service, which fills over eight million prescriptions a year, one can easily see that the vast majority of prescriptions address similar, if not the same, problems. The AARP list for 1991 includes:

1. Cardizem (for treatment of cardiac difficulties)
2. Furosemide/generic for Lasix (a diuretic that causes the kidneys to excrete more water)
3. Tenormin (for heart and blood pressure)

4. Digoxin/generic for Lanoxin (used to stabilize heart contractions)
5. Dipyridamole/generic for Persantine (basically used for high blood pressure, as well as an adjunct to surgical procedures)
6. Capoten (heart/blood pressure)
7. Triamterene/Hydrochlorothiazide/generic for Dyazide (a diuretic for the treatment of high blood pressure)
8. Mevacor (This is a new drug used for lowering cholesterol)
9. Premarin (for osteoporosis/menopause)
10. KCL (tablet form)/generic for Slow-K/potassium/ Vitamin K (used for potassium replacement, usually in conjunction with a diuretic).

According to Steve Grote at the AARP Pharmacy Service, other top prescriptions include a Ventolin and proventil inhaler that's used for emphysema and asthma; Zantac, for ulcers; and Micronase, which diabetics use to affect their blood-sugar level.

From reading about medications and older people, I had assumed that a vast number of medications given to older people addressed mood and were treatment for depression or anxiety. I had the impression that these drugs were the most overused and abused drugs prescribed to older people. I understood that older women particularly were given tranquilizers to treat their symptoms of nervousness, restlessness, or depression instead of being given an appropriate diagnosis.

Hugo Koch at the National Center for Health Statistics said that when he began his comprehensive study of 135 million prescriptions, he, too, hypothesized that the elderly—and most particularly older women—were given excessive amounts of tranquilizers, sedatives, and other psychotropic drugs. But when all the data was compiled, the list of the top twenty-five drugs ordered or provided for patients seventy-five and older during office visits didn't contain one single tranquilizer or psychotropic drug.

"It's mythology that we're overdosing our ambulatory elderly with tranquilizers," Mr. Koch said in an interview. "The use of minor tranquilizers, like Valium, can be seen in only 6 percent of all the visits—which amounts to about fifty-seven tranquilizers per one thousand visits." On the other hand, the Public Citizen Health Research Group has found that the most dangerously overused kinds of drugs within the larger category of psychotropic/mind-affecting drugs are minor tranquilizers or antidepressants such as Valium, Librium, Xanax, Tranxene, the less used barbiturates (such as Nembutal/phenobarbital or Seconal), and antipsychotic drugs, major tranquilizers such as Haldol, Thorazine, Mellaril, Stelazine, and Prolixin. They've found that older adults are prescribed over one-third of all minor and major tranquilizers and antidepressants. In addition, more than half of all prescriptions for sleeping pills are filled by older adults.

View Based on Nursing Home Reality

If older people in the community are being overdosed with tranquilizers and sedatives, then residents of nursing homes and hospitals are being absolutely inundated by them. Profiles on this overdosing are based on actual data from inpatient treatment in hospitals and nursing homes, where it's always been easier to give a patient a tranquilizer or an antidepressant than to deal with his anxiety or emotional upset. Those data show that almost one-third of all residents in long-term care institutions receive between eight and sixteen drugs daily. Some studies have shown that residents routinely receive between twelve and sixteen drugs daily. In these nursing-care facilities, some *one out of four of the top twenty-five drugs are sedatives, hypnotics, or psychotropic drugs*. According to a study of physicians prescribing patterns in skilled nursing facilities in 1976, *more than half* of nursing-home residents received psychotropic drugs. An earlier study showed that only two tranquilizers, Librium and Valium, were in the top ten most frequently dispensed drugs in nursing homes.

According to Dr. Peter Lamy at the University of Maryland, the top six categories of drugs used in nursing homes, accounting for 70 percent of all their prescriptions, were psychotropics, cardiovascular drugs, laxatives, analgesics, vitamins, and diuretics.

Like many other institutions, nursing homes fall into the habit of using chemicals as a way of maintaining order and control in the population. There are, however, some less despicable reasons for the heavy use of medicines in nursing homes. Many residents of nursing homes and hospitals are struggling with life-threatening or sanity-threatening diseases. Many drugs that are given to nursing-home patients are involved in their crisis interventions, emergency treatment, and long-term maintenance. Those drugs—which may include cancer chemotherapy, insulin, and some antihypertensives, and a good number of psychotropics that are closely monitored by medical staffs—do indicate serious levels of illness. Nevertheless, the use of multiple drugs seems almost always to lead to the necessity of more drugs, rather than fewer. Dr. James Cooper and others who have studied nursing-home prescribing patterns assert that most nursing-home patients could have their medicines cut in half with no adverse effects.

Since the study of physicians' prescribing patterns in nursing homes in 1976, there have been government efforts to reduce drug use in these facilities. Federal standards caution that use of more than 6.2 drugs per patient per day indicates that there may be problems in drug prescribing for federally financed (Medicare) patients. The federal government now mandates that a pharmacist must review the drug regimens of all patients in nursing homes that receive federal money. Most of the elderly, however, are not in nursing homes, and yet their illnesses and drug regimens are often just as complicated as those of their nursing-home counterparts. According to Dr. Lamy, for every resident in a nursing home, there are four elderly people of equal disability being cared for at home. There is still no formal mechanism for reimbursement, however, to provide for a pharmacist to monitor their drug regimens, or to report possible problems to the physicians who prescribe them.

Drugs Used in Home Health Care

No good statistics seem to be available on drug use in home health care—where people are visited and treated often by state, county, or community doctors and nurses. This mode of treatment will probably continue to increase as the older population grows—and as less space is available in hospitals and nursing homes for long-term treatment.

According to Dr. Lamy, "anecdotal evidence seems to indicate that drug use is high [in home health care], and the size per prescription is higher than what has been previously experienced, perhaps to save the patient money." Also, he says, more narcotics and anti-anxiety drugs are being used for home-care patients than for people who live in the community or in nursing homes. From research in a day treatment center, Dr. Lamy and his colleagues found that there was a high use of "convenience" drugs—drugs not correlated to the patients' needs but given instead for the convenience of the staff. Nonprescription drugs also seemed to be prescribed liberally and used even more widely by the elderly. Additionally, many drugs were prescribed on an "as needed" basis, which makes the monitoring of drug effects extremely difficult.

WHEN YOUR DOCTOR WRITES A
PRESCRIPTION

Under normal circumstances, when your doctor writes a prescription for you, she has chosen a medication from one of a group of drugs used to treat your condition. Many factors go into making that choice, including your medical history, your age, height, and weight. Doctors describe their decision-making process in different ways.

"One of the cautions that goes through my mind is knowing that it's often better to take them off a medication than to put them on one," says Dr. John Rowe of Mount Sinai Medical Center. "Basically, when I write a prescription for an older person, three things go through my mind. The first is their drug-age interaction. I wonder, how will this drug work in the body of this older person? The second thought is the drug-disease interaction. I want to treat this patient's blood pressure, but what effect will it have on her in other ways? What other problems does this person have? The third thing is the drug–drug interaction. What other medications is this person taking? Those are the three things that help me, and they're easy to remember."

Dr. Michael Freedman, director of the Division of Geriatrics at New York University Medical Center in New York City, says that one of the first questions he asks himself is, "Does the person need this medicine?"

"I always wonder whether the illness is worse than the treatment that I have available," he says. "And then I wonder whether there's another way I can treat this patient other than giving him or her a prescription that is equally effective. For instance, can I get a mildly diabetic person to lose weight?

"Another big consideration is 'Will the patient accept anything *but* a prescription?' Given who this patient is, what he does, and what other medications he's taking, will he be able to take this medicine and take it the way he's supposed to? Will he be able to follow the instructions and take it every three hours?

"The bottom line is that I wonder whether the patient will get better and feel better if I give him this medicine, or whether there is any other way of doing it."

Unfortunately, says Dr. Freedman, doctors too often bow to the pressure of their patients and write more prescriptions than they believe they should. Constraints of time, energy, and money add to the pressure. The system also beats down doctors, he said, referring to a recent article in the *New England Journal of Medicine* written by a doctor in western Massachusetts who had to accept Medicare assignments. Like others, this doctor has to make enough money to pay for her office overhead as well as the rising premiums of her malpractice insurance. At twenty-three dollars a visit from Medicare, she figured that she has to move people out of her office every ten minutes in order to meet her expenses. She doesn't have time to explain anything to them. "In circumstances like that," says Dr. Freedman, "doctors find themselves saying, 'You came in for a pill? Here's a pill!' They don't have time to think about the quality of life in the elderly or what those medications can do to affect that quality."

Undermedicating

Interestingly enough, painkillers are one kind of medication that doctors may not prescribe enough of when patients need them. Doctors tend to underdose painkillers, and patients tend not to take them as directed.

If you have been prescribed a painkiller by your doctor, don't wait for the pain to be intense before you take pain medication for it. If you're taking a mild analgesic, it may not work if your pain level is extremely high. Sometimes you might avoid taking these medications because you're afraid of becoming addicted to them, or perhaps you're stoic and think that taking the medicine is exhibiting weakness. But if you wait too long, the medicine may not be effective. Also, the pain might keep you from moving around, coughing, or breathing deeply. For those reasons, especially after surgery, it's better to take the medicine instead of letting your pain threshold get too high. By taking the medicine as it's prescribed, and thereby being able to move, breathe, and cough freely, you'll get better faster.

Some doctors may also underprescribe when it comes to antidepressants. Some studies indicate that 20 percent of the elderly may suffer from depression, and as many as 90 percent of these cases may go unrecognized. According to Madeline Feinberg, a pharmacist and director of the Elder-Health Program at the University of Maryland at Baltimore, it's very sad when older people who could be treated successfully with an antidepressant never have any recognition of their condition. "Another thing that happens is that the symptoms are misdiagnosed and the patient ends up with a drug for anxiety or insomnia instead of one targeted for depression," says Ms. Feinberg. "Then, if an antidepressant is given, and in very cautious doses, there may be fear of increasing the dose due to the possibility of side effects occurring, and the patient remains undertreated."

Overmedicating

Often longstanding prescriptions simply aren't needed. The Public Citizen Health Research Group, headed by Dr. Sidney Wolfe, estimates that at least two-thirds of the prescriptions filled by older adults are: 1) given in unnecessarily high doses that cause extra risks without extra benefits, 2) unnecessarily dangerous because a less dangerous drug is available that would be equally beneficial, or 3) not needed at all because they are not the solution for the patient's problem. That research group and its medical consultants also assert that at least 104 of the 287 most commonly prescribed drugs for older adults should not be used by older adults because safer or more effective alternative drugs are available.

At the Coffey Geriatric Clinic at Mount Sinai Hospital in New York City, the interdisciplinary staff slowly weans patients from the medications that can be discontinued without any harmful effects. These can include common medications that people might not even think to mention or review, let alone eliminate, from their daily consumption. These include laxatives, sedatives, some vitamins, hypnotics, tranquilizers, some cardiac drugs, and some seizure drugs.

Many prescriptions, like laxatives—which are the single most frequently used class of drugs in long-term care institutions—are given almost automatically, when natural alternatives can be far more effective and produce fewer side effects. Here are some observations that the interdisciplinary teams at Mount Sinai's geriatric clinic have made on the elimination of unnecessary drugs:

LAXATIVES Some of you may be on as many as four different laxatives. If staff members took your dietary history, they would probably find out that you're not getting enough water or enough bran. What you need isn't a prescription for a laxative. They'll tell you that what you need is water, bran, spinach, applesauce, and roughage.

SEDATIVES, HYPNOTICS, OR DAYTIME TRANQUILIZERS Almost 90 percent of the sleeping pills prescribed could be eliminated, according to Dr. Charles Herrera, a sleep specialist at Mount Sinai. Sleeping pills such as Dalmane, Noludar, Restoril, Halcion, and tranquilizers like Xanax and Valium can be extremely problematic for any older person. You may wake up drowsy and need to go to the bathroom, but you're so sedated that you fall down and end up with a hip fracture. Or you may have mental confusion that appears to be dementia. If you have trouble sleeping at night, eliminate your day-time naps. Try getting up at the same time every morning, whether or not you've slept soundly. Eat well and take a brisk walk during the day. If you wake up in the night, don't fret. Get out a good book or watch TV. You'll fall asleep again when you get tired.

CARDIAC DRUGSIf you had a heart incident twenty years ago, you may have been on digoxin all that time. Doctors at Mount Sinai say that they're not even sure why digoxin was originally prescribed, but they see people who have been taking it for twenty years. If you fall into this category, ask your doctor if you still need the drug. It may well be that you don't.

SEIZURE DRUGSIf your arm shook thirty years ago, you may still be on medication for that complaint. You may be afraid that you'll have a seizure without the medication, but it may well be that it is entirely extraneous. Talk to your doctor. The worst thing you'll find out is that you still need the drug to control seizures.

NUTRITIONAL SUPPLEMENTSIf you go into the Coffey Clinic and you're taking megadoses of vitamins, they'll tell you that megadoses can be very damaging. In the right doses, vitamins A and D can be helpful, they say, but too much can make you crazy. Too much selenium can be toxic to the liver.

"The fact is that a large segment of the population doesn't need the medicine they use," says pharmacist Randall Wright. "Doctors have to be aware that there are other ways of giving medicine than two, three, or four times a day. But it's hard to teach people to do things differently from the way they were taught. In my opinion, many problems now are directly caused by too much high blood pressure medicine. If the patient is dieting and exercising, and managing stress under the doctor's direction, the doctor could say, 'Here are some pills. Take them two or three times a week.' In many cases, this would be an appropriate dosage.

"There's talk about why there's all this overmedication," says Wright, who finds that he spends a great deal of time helping patients help their doctors to wean them from their drugs. "It's simple. Physicians and pharmacists handle medicine too casually. They write two or three prescriptions without a thought. Why should patients have a different attitude about them? Why shouldn't they be careless? It's a state of carelessness gone into a state of recklessness.

"The solution is for health-care professionals to set a better example with the use of medicines and for the patient to be made aware that health in a bottle of pills is just not there. Medications can be an incredible help, but they don't provide total health. Patients need to lose weight, exercise, or take care of themselves differently when their doctors tell them to. Most are more than willing."

CHAPTER 4

Taking Command of Your Prescriptions

"Age only matters when one is aging. Now that I have
arrived at a great age, I might as well be twenty."
—PABLO PICASSO

A doctor who writes you a prescription is handing you
a responsibility. You're the one in charge of your medication. Are you ready to be the manager? Do you feel
well coached about what you're doing?

To be an informed consumer, your most important
task is to learn the fundamentals. There's no FDA requirement that written instructions and warnings be
given with a prescribed medication, so you must find
out this information for yourself.*

Start at the beginning. When you get a prescription,
look at it. Can you read it? Is it legible? Half of the
pharmacists who responded to a poll by the *American
Druggist* said that they'd made errors in dispensing
drugs because of doctors' sloppy writing. If you can't
read the writing on your prescription, whether it's your
eyes or the handwriting, ask the doctor or nurse to print
or type the words on the prescription right under or over
the hieroglyphics. Make sure the name of the drug is
clear. Repeat it and write it down for yourself if necessary. Also write down what it's for. If, for instance,
it's Maalox, and your doctor tells you it's for your stomach, write down ''Maalox—antacid for stomach upset.''

*At the end of the book, we've included a list of questions for you to
ask about your prescriptions when you visit your health-care specialist.

Spell it out. He might be saying Maalox, but if it sounds like "Marax" to you and you don't spell it out, you might end up with a bronchodilator instead of an antacid. A lot of drugs look alike and sound alike, and you don't want to fall victim to medication errors because you were given a sedative called Haldol instead of a male hormone called Halotestin. Nor would you want to have the pharmacist mistake Terfonyl for Tofranil. The first is a sulfonamide, and the second is an antidepressant.

Once you've established the name of the medicine, ask your doctor what it is supposed to do for you, how it will make you feel, and how it will interact with your other medications. Take responsibility. When you don't know, ask questions. Never be afraid of sounding stupid.

"Is this medicine necessary?"

"What will it do for me?"

"How is it supposed to work?"

"What are the side effects?"

"Are there alternatives to this medicine that would be better for me?"

"Should I take it with food or liquids or on an empty stomach?"

"Are there any foods I should avoid?" (Some medicines can't be taken with certain foods and liquids. See more in chapter 8.)

Grace Landis (who happens to be my mother) is a good example of an informed consumer. A vital seventy-four-year-old who works as a volunteer at her local art museum, she regularly attends the symphony, reads voraciously, and travels extensively. She has always taken it upon herself to know all about the medicine she's taking. Although she had a hysterectomy because of cervical cancer some sixteen years ago and had a hip replacement four years ago, her health is generally good.

"When I get a prescription, I ask my doctor what it is and why he's giving it to me," she says. "I also ask if there are any side effects I should watch for. I check with my pharmacist whether to take it with food or away from food. I know, for instance, that if I'm taking a tetracycline, I should not eat cheese.

"I think it's terrible not to be told these things automatically, but I also think that knowing what you're taking and as much as you can about it is part of the responsibility of a patient.

"When I have a prescription I haven't had before, I look it up in *The Physicians' Desk Reference*, James Long's *Essential Guide to Prescription Drugs*, or *The Merck Manual*," she says. "I look up side effects and what foods should or should not be taken with this medication.

"After my hip surgery, I happened to hear someone say that you need to go on an antibiotic when you have dental work done because of having a foreign body [the artificial hip] in your body. They said that otherwise, just because of the dental work, you can get a serious infection that could cause a lot of trouble with the surgery. I asked my surgeon about it during a follow-up visit, and he said yes, that I should take an antibiotic when I have dental work done. I asked him why I hadn't been told that, and he said it was not a routine thing, but that since I'd asked, he thought it was a good idea. When I talked to my dentist about it, he was adamant that I have the antibiotic. He says it's a must for anyone with anything artificial in the body.

"He recently gave me a new prescription for an antibiotic [erythromycin]. I keep that on hand, and I always take it with me if I go to Europe or on a trip. If I'm having dental work, I take one antibiotic four times a day for three days, starting twenty-four hours before my appointment.

"The most recent medicine I was given is Corgard. It's a beta-blocker for hypertension and to help prevent strokes. I've been on it for three or four years—one tablet once a day, and I never miss it. I've made my sisters ask their doctors about it because they've had hypertension longer than me. My doctor started me on one-fourth tablet and then slowly increased it to one tablet.

"I saw a recent television interview where a doctor tried to cut a pill in half with a pill cutter. He showed that you just can't do it. He said that companies should make pills one-quarter or one-half strength for older people, because when you cut it, you're either not getting half or you're getting more than half!"

It's always important to ask your doctor about the side effects of the medication you're receiving because all medications have side effects—even if they're minor and even if they don't happen to you. Also ask your doctor whether there are any effects the medication may have that are *not* intended. Knowing about potential side effects can save you time and money. For instance, if you know a stomachache is an expected side effect of a particular medicine, when you get one, you'll eat a cracker instead of calling the doctor. If you know that an *unintended* side effect is vomiting and nausea, you'll know that you're not just getting the flu if you have this reaction, and you'll call your doctor immediately.

If your physician says he doesn't like to tell a patient about side effects because he doesn't want the patient to be anxious or to develop symptoms that he otherwise might not have, tell him that there is no scientific evidence that if you give people more information they get more symptoms. Tell him that you want to know about any potential problems.

Many people look up their prescriptions in medical references that list, in easy-to-read type, the possible side effects or adverse reactions that have been reported on various drugs on the market. Some of this information sounds alarming, making the side effects sound worse than the disease itself. Remember, however, that not everyone has the side effects, and some of the adverse side effects happen only to one in ten or twenty thousand people. If you use a reference book and learn something your doctor, dentist, nurse, or pharmacist didn't mention, call one of them about it.

"IT'S ALL GREEK TO ME"

When you receive your prescription from the doctor, it's important to make sure that you understand it. The symbols on your prescriptions may look as if they're written in a foreign language; many are, in fact, abbreviated Latin words, left over from the days when doctors wrote prescriptions in Latin. Don't try to make sense out of them in English, and don't be intimidated by them. They're easy to translate—and it's important that you do so in order to clarify when and how often you should take your medication.

On the prescription it may say *TID*, *QID*, *Topical*, *Gtts*, or any number of other symbols you don't understand. These are Latin terms that give you critical information about when to take your medicine. The *Q* stands for "quarterly," the *D* for "*diem,*" or day. *Bid* is short for "*Bis in die*"—twice a day. Symbols for *when* to take the medicine are translated as follows:

BID—Two times a day	stat—At once, first dose
TID—Three times a day	
QID—Four times a day	x—Times
QOD—Every other day	qhs—At hour of sleep
QD—Daily	qlh—Every hour
h—Hourly	q2h—Every two hours
ac—Before meals	q3h—Every three hours
pc—After meals	
AM—Morning	q4h—Every four hours
PM—Evening	
prn—As needed	ut dict—As directed

Directions on your prescription tell you the root of administration as well. They tell you what form this medicine comes in (tablets, capsules, liquid, suppositories, or ointments) and how it should be taken. Is it taken by mouth or is it put in the rectum? Does it go in your eyes or on your skin? Don't laugh! Sometimes you really *don't* know the difference unless you're told what part of the body it goes into. Symbols for *how* to take the medicine are translated as follows:

A2—Both ears	5 ml—One teaspoon
AD—Right ear	O—One pint
AL—Left ear	O2—Both eyes
cc—Cubic centimeter	OD—Right eye
cap—Capsule	OL—Left eye
ext—For external use	OS—Left eye
gtts—Drops	sol—Solution
gutta—Drop	ss—Half unit
OU—Each eye	susp—Suspension
po—By mouth	tab—Tablet
pr—By rectum	top—Apply topically
IV—Intravenous	ung or
IM—Intramuscular	ungt—Ointment
s.c.—Subcutaneously	sl—Under the
ml—Milliliter (Thirty milliliters equal one ounce)	tongue

If a medication is to be used for the eyes, it should be clearly labeled "For Ophthalmic Use Only." If it doesn't say anything about "Ophthalmic Use," it shouldn't be used in the eyes. Nurses have all too often seen patients who were given a prescription for bacitracin ophthalmic ointment instead put the regular bacitracin ointment they have in their cupboard in their eyes. Don't do this. It's the same medicine, but the ointment for your eyes is sterile, and the one for your skin isn't.

If you put skin ointment in your eyes, it can be damaging.

"Topical Use Only" means that you should use this medicine only on the *outside* of your body.

Certain kinds of vaginal creams should be used outside on the labia only. If you are getting some vaginal cream, make sure to ask your doctor whether or not you can put it inside your vagina as well as outside it. Ask him to tell you where you should put it and where you shouldn't put it.

Suppositories are *not* to be swallowed. They go up the rectum if they're rectal suppositories or up the vagina if they're vaginal suppositories. *Ask* for directions.

Don't feel silly asking the doctor "How do I take this medicine?" There are a number of different avenues besides swallowing. It might be important, for instance, for you to dissolve a pill under your tongue instead of swallowing it. Someone with chest pains will probably be directed to put her nitroglycerin tablet under the tongue to dissolve *sublingually*. That's because those veins under your tongue lead right into your vascular system, so when the nitroglycerin dissolves there, it gets absorbed directly into the bloodstream.

If you are given a nitropatch, you need to know *where* it goes on your chest. Does it go closer to the heart or to the middle of the chest? When you wear a nitropatch, the nitroglycerin is absorbed through the skin, so you need to know how long to leave on the patch. It should not be left on indefinitely.

Ask *what time of day* it's best to take your medicine. If you're on a diuretic, for instance, ask your doctor whether you should take it in the morning or in the evening. Usually doctors recommend that you take your diuretic in the morning because if you take it in the evening, you're apt to be up all night going to the bathroom. Also, if you're going back and forth from the bathroom at night, you increase your chances of a fall.

Also ask, *Should I add anything to my diet or avoid any foods or beverages because of this medication?* For example, if you're on certain diuretics, you might need to eat food that's high in potassium because the diuretic robs you of potassium. With these diuretics, the doctor may recommend that you eat a banana (or a number of other foods high in potassium) every time you take the pill. On the other hand, there are some diuretics that are potassium-sparing, so if you changed diuretics and you still were eating a banana a day, you could overload your system with potassium—which could cause you cardiac problems. In some cases, you may need to take vitamin or mineral supplements to replace nutrients lost because of the effects of the medication. Some drugs should *never* be taken on an empty stomach, and others require that you avoid certain foods because of their interaction with the drug.

Sometimes your prescription will have a *c* or an *s* written on it—*c* means "with," and *s* means "without." Be alert to these symbols, and make sure to ask.

LIFE-STYLE CHANGES

Another important question you should ask: *Is there any alteration of my daily routine I should consider* because of this medication? If you're taking any medicines that affect coordination, reaction time, alertness, or vision, you'll need to know from your doctor whether you should stop driving or doing certain activities.

Dilantin for seizure disorders, major tranquilizers for psychosis, minor tranquilizers for anxiety, and barbiturates, hypnotics, or sedatives for sleep can dramatically affect your alertness and reaction time. Remember that you could lose a finger on the drill or under a knife if you don't have your normal coordination and quick reaction time.

Finding out what the possible side effects of a drug are might make you decide, for instance, not to drive the tractor or to fix the furnace right now because you know you won't be as alert as usual. Knowing what to expect will help you make the necessary adjustments and alterations to avoid hazards.

If you are outdoors quite a bit, or if it's summertime, ask your doctor, nurse, or pharmacist about your exposure to sunlight while you're on a particular medication. Some drugs can make you more sensitive to sunlight and thus cause you to sunburn very easily.

If you were going to ask only one question about your prescription, that question should be, *Is there anything I need to change in my life-style, be aware of, or not do when I take this drug?* By asking this question, you're alerting the physician that you're an aware consumer who really wants this information. It means that you can be a better patient because you have an understanding of what to look for and know to report information to your doctor more quickly. You have an understanding of how you can best help the medicine help you.

Steer Clear of Medical Jargon

If your doctor explains what to do in medical jargon and you don't understand what she's saying, ask her to tell you again, in plain English. Don't be embarrassed if you don't know what a health-care professional is talking about and don't be intimidated if anyone acts condescending or acts as if you should know exactly what is being said. A good doctor wants you to take your medications properly. Sometimes a doctor has to be reminded that you haven't been to medical school, nor are you a pharmacist, so there's some fundamental information that may take a few extra minutes for you to learn. It's vital that you know just what to do and how to do it, because, after all, you are the one in charge of making sure that this medicine is properly administered.

If you don't hear the instructions properly, you may not want to admit that fact. Admit it. Ask to be told again, loudly, or have it written down for you, or both.

If you can't see what is written down for you to read about your medication—including the instructions—ask your doctor or nurse to write it in large print. If they do write it in large print and you still can't read it, tell them. Ask them to help you figure out what to do about it.

If for any reason you decide not to fill your prescription or take the medication as prescribed, inform your doctor of your decision before you leave his office or after you've made the decision at home. If you're not going to fill the prescription, you should know the possible alternatives you have, or the doctor's opinion about the consequences of that decision.

WHERE SHOULD YOU GET YOUR PRESCRIPTION FILLED?

Picking a good pharmacist and a good pharmacy can be just as important as picking a good doctor. A good pharmacist is a gold mine of information. He's a scientifically trained professional who can act as your advisor on practical and technical matters relating to your medications. Unless you have a very unusual doctor, your pharmacist will know a great deal more about the medicines you're on than your doctor does. Medications are the pharmacist's lifework. You might as well be one of the people to benefit from his knowledge.

Over the years, the role of the pharmacist has changed. Pharmacists are no longer involved only in the dispensing of drugs. Now they're much more involved in drug information and monitoring, both on an individual patient basis and on a total institutional basis.

Pharmacists in hospitals, for instance, review how the drugs are used within the institution, how they're prescribed, why they're prescribed, how they're administered, and how they're followed up for adverse drug reactions as well as for positive reactions. They find out whether or not the drug was effective, and why. Good pharmacists are interested in your health and well-being. Most good pharmacists see their work on your behalf as an important part of their role as health-care professionals in the community.

It's a good idea to buy all your prescription and non-prescription drugs from the same pharmacy. During the course of my research on this book, I found a number of pharmacies in small towns where the pharmacists told their clients that if they weren't going to buy *all* their prescriptions from them, then they didn't want them to buy any. These pharmacists knew that they would lose some business from such a demand, but they believed firmly that it was in their customers' best interests.

"I don't want to play that game with your health," says Barry Sarvis, owner of his own pharmacy in Manhattan, Kansas. "Either I do all of them or I don't want to do them at all. Otherwise, I won't know your whole health picture. Some people call and go to five different drugstores looking for the best price. They'll call up and ask, 'How much is so and so?' They'll get different prescriptions from different doctors and different drug stores, and no one has the whole list of what they're doing. That's just an accident waiting to happen."

Standing behind the counter in his large, well-lit pharmacy, Barry Sarvis talks personally with each customer about every prescription he fills. He pulls out the record he keeps on each customer every time he fills a new prescription. He looks at what the person is taking, asks him about his life and health, and quite clearly serves as a health counselor, if not a personal counselor, to the young and old people who come into his store.

Even in large cities, it's possible to find a drugstore where the pharmacist will develop a relationship with you, talk to you about your medicines, and keep tabs on your prescriptions. Shop around. Find one who is willing to spend the time to get to know you and to help you with your medicines. Many pharmacists take an interest in doing more than just selling their products. When you're looking for the right place to buy your drugs, ask the pharmacist if he will keep a list of all the drugs you're taking, including your nonprescription drugs. Ask if he is willing to keep track of drug interactions and to help you avoid drugs that, if taken together, might be harmful to you. Also ask if he would intervene on your behalf by calling your doctor if he noticed any prescription that could cause you harm.

Responsible pharmacists will keep a record of your allergies and earlier drug reactions. They'll write down your medications and will check new prescriptions against that list. Today quite a few pharmacies have all the information about your prescriptions in a computerized system. This works to your advantage because it's easy for the pharmacist to check your new prescriptions' interactive effects with the old medicines you're taking. You should also check with your pharmacist before buying any over-the-counter drugs, and ask that OTCs are kept as part of your record.

It might be tempting to pick up a nonprescription drug in a grocery store, but if, for instance, you wanted to pick up a bottle of Advil, there's no one in the grocery store to tell you that this is a potent drug. A stock boy or a grocer can't tell you how Advil will interact with your particular condition or with the other medicines you're taking.

Intervention on Your Behalf

Your pharmacist can be one of your best allies when it comes to handling your medications properly. If you hand your pharmacist a prescription, for instance, that is clearly contradictory to the other medicines you're on, he or she can call your doctor and ask about it. The pharmacist doesn't have the power to *change* your prescription, but she does have the authority to tell the doctor that this is a dangerous combination. Most likely, the doctor would respond by changing the prescription. If not, the pharmacist can tell your doctor that she is advising you not to take it. In an extreme case, your pharmacist may tell the doctor that she's making note of what the doctor is saying, will advise the patient of her own opinion, and make the situation a matter of record.

According to the Elder-Health program at the University of Maryland School of Pharmacy, your pharmacist can provide other services as well. These include:

- Notifying you when a refill is due. This can be very important because when a drug has been prescribed for a chronic disease, it's important not to interrupt treatment.
- Typing the labels on your prescription bottle in large print if the regular print is too small for you to read.
- Discussing with you the correct ways to take your prescriptions. Your pharmacist should know all the answers to questions about how, when, and how much medicine is to be taken, what side effects and other responses to expect from the medicine, what to avoid or change when it comes to food and activity and your medicine, and how to store your medications.
- Giving you containers you can easily open. (Make sure you try to open the container while you're still at the pharmacy. If you can't get the top off, ask for

a non-childproof container. Then make sure to keep
it away from any grandchildren in your house.)
- Giving you written information on your medication
  when it has been supplied to him by the drug company.
- Giving you written reminders, calendars, or other
  materials to help you take your medicine correctly.

Many times, having a dialogue with your pharmacist
can make a world of difference in your sense of confidence about your medications. He can explain the
meaning of the drug to you and help you know what to
expect at various stages. If, for instance, you have a
urinary infection and you're taking a medication that
turns your urine red, you may think you're bleeding and
quit taking the medicine. Naturally, your infection will
get worse in that case and you'll get sicker. In reality,
the medicine was doing exactly what it was predicted
to do, but nobody told you about it.

By advising you how to manage your medications
effectively and consistently, your pharmacist will be
helping you to cut your overall medical costs. Without
false alarms or adverse reactions that occur from misusing medications, you'll pay fewer doctors' bills and
avoid trips to emergency rooms and to the hospital.
Another important economic function your pharmacists
can fulfill is to help you cut costs by substituting generic
drugs for more expensive brand name drugs when
they're appropriate.

GENERIC DRUGS

If you've wondered what, exactly, a generic drug is, it's
simply a replication of a brand name drug that's generally less expensive than its trademark equivalent. The
generic name of a drug is also called the ''official'' or
''nonproprietary'' name, which is usually descriptive of

the chemical composition or class of the drug. A generic name is assigned to each drug in the early stages of its development and, like other drugs, it is identified in three different ways:

- By its trade or brand name, which is invented by the drug company that develops and produces it. (This name is generally capitalized, with the trademark symbol after the name.)
- By its more commonly used name, which is its generic name, usually a shorter version of the chemical name.
- By its specific chemical name, which describes the chemical composition of the drug. (Also not capitalized.)

Most consumers know the original brand names of drugs. For instance, most of us know the name Librium, the original drug, but not the generic name, chlordiazepoxide hydrochloride. The brand name sometimes refers to a particular combination of drugs but doesn't necessarily relate to the chemical name. Aspirin, for instance, is a generic name, while Bayer is a brand name. The *chemical* name for aspirin is acetylsalicylic acid. The relationship of the generic to the brand name is similar to that between the words *mayonnaise* and *Hellmans'*.

For consumers, the most significant difference between generic drugs and brand name drugs is that generics cost much less. A survey by the Federal Trade Commission in 1985 revealed that the sale of generic drugs during the previous year had resulted in $130 to $236 million in savings to the American consumer. At that time, Secretary of Health and Human Services Margaret Heckler estimated that if the ten most frequently prescribed prescriptions in 1981 had been filled with generic equivalents, American consumers would have saved $500 million. She pointed out that the average cost of generic equivalents was approximately half the cost of brand name prescriptions.

For many people, this savings can be of critical importance. Sara and Bill Hunter found, for instance, that when they received a bill for Sara's mother from the nursing home, Sara's mother had been charged for two orders of twenty ten-milligram Librium at fifteen dollars each. Since Sara's mother receives twenty-five dollars a month of her own social security for all her expenses—everything from medication to toothpaste—her funds for a month and a half had been consumed merely by the expense of the Librium.

"I asked the pharmacist, 'What's a substitute for Librium?' " says Bill. "He told me that the generic form of Librium [chlordiazepoxide hydrochloride] is the same and that a one-hundred-tablet bottle is $6.95. That will last her three and a half months!"

The reason brand name drugs cost the consumer so much more than generics is that it costs brand name manufacturers a great deal more money to create and market the original drug than it does for the generic company to copy it. In 1986, it was estimated that a pharmaceutical company would spend $100 million to conduct the studies required by the FDA to bring one drug to the market *after* developing it in the laboratory animals. It cost another $100 million to advertise and promote it to physicians.

When a new drug is developed, the manufacturer sells it under an exclusive patent for a number of years (which varies from drug to drug) until the patent expires. During that time, only the manufacturer who holds the patent can sell the drug, which it markets under a brand name. For example, until recently, only Hoffman La Roche Pharmaceuticals could sell Valium, the original trade name for diazepam, under the name Valium. When the patent expired, however, the originator no longer had the exclusive right to produce the product. Any firm can theoretically produce and market the drug under the generic name or a new brand name (the original manufacturer retains exclusive use of the original brand name).

Beyond production and marketing costs, the only expense a company producing a generic has is to prove to the government that its product is the *bioequivalent* of the trade name drug. This means that they have to prove that the generic drug behaves the same way in the body as the original drug.

Are Generics as Good?
The Federal Food and Drug Administration (FDA) evaluates each generic drug in terms of its bioequivalency. While it may look different from the original drug in shape, size, and color, the generic medicine has to behave the same way in the body as the original. It also has to have the identical amount of the active ingredients of the drug and be in the same dosage form. The generic drugs are tested for bioequivalence on human beings who consume them and then have their blood level measured to determine the amount of the active chemical in their blood. The FDA will accept as bioequivalent a difference of plus or minus 20 percent from the original drug. Pharmacists say this is reasonable given the fact that within any product there can be batch-to-batch variability, which is clinically insignificant. Certainly there is at least that much variability in the bodies of the patients who take the drugs as well. For drugs that are more erratically absorbed, such as psychotropic drugs, the FDA allows a 30 percent plus or minus difference for bioequivalency.

Some critics say that this variability is too flexible a standard. The Pharmaceutical Manufacturers Association, for instance, maintains that the bioequivalency standards are too inexact. They also say that there are differences in the care with which the drugs are made, the formula, the inactive ingredients, and the rate at which the tablet dissolves, among other things. Some physicians also have strong feelings against generics, saying that they prefer the consistency of the brands with which they are familiar. Others point to the 1984 Hatch-Waxman Act (the Drug Price Competition and Patent Term Restoration Act, which made it possible for generic companies to produce drugs without the lengthy safety-and-effectiveness approval process needed in the past) as a sign that quality controls in generic manufacturing are not sufficiently uniform to assure therapeutic equivalence. (This process was shortened so long as the drugs are bioequivalent to the brand name drugs that are already considered safe and effective.)

Many consumer groups and physicians, however, say that these arguments are self-serving, proprietary matters, and that the arguments against generics aren't convincing. Some say that one of the main sentiments against generics is the fear that they will cut into the profits of leading pharmaceutical companies, lower their incentive to develop new products, and force them to reduce their research budgets—which last year totaled $4 billion. (Total sales of the pharmaceutical industry reached $17.5 billion in 1986 and were expected to jump to $24.3 billion by 1990, according to the Stanford Research Institute.)

In the meantime, the FDA and many consumer groups, including the American Association of Retired Persons (AARP), maintain that generics are as safe, effective, and equivalent therapeutically as brand name drugs. They point out that the 80 percent of older people who pay for their prescriptions out of their own pockets can benefit greatly from the savings. Some insurance companies and prescription drug benefit plans obviously think that generics are safe because they require the pharmacist to provide patients with generic drugs when they're available. It's not unusual for certain insurance companies to refuse reimbursement unless the lowest-cost drug has been provided. Sometimes, when a pharmacist would prefer not to give a generic, this puts him under pressure to do so, or to collect the difference from the patients.

Should Consumers Buy Generics?

If you're starting a new medication, you should ask your pharmacist if it's available generically. Your pharmacist will have a list of generic products found to be therapeutically equivalent by the FDA and your state. Refer to it. If, for instance, you have a prescription for methyldopa and you're going to be taking one hundred pills a month for the rest of your life, it makes sense to spend 50 or 60 percent less for them if you can.

You don't have to worry about the quality of the generics your pharmacist will stock. Often the term "generic" conjures up the image of a mom-and-pop bathtub business or a very small plant where workers file into a small basement to fill capsules by hand. This is not the case. "The bathtub drugs and the schlock-house generics are a thing of the past," one pharmacist told me. "Today some 90 percent of the generics are produced by major drug firms in the country, many being the well-known manufacturers of brand name drugs." Parke-Davis has a generic line, for instance, as does Squibb. Other major generic companies were also manufacturers for major companies under trade labels before, and now have simply branched out on their own. Certain smaller generic companies are owned by large pharmaceutical concerns. Pharmacists seem to agree that as a rule, the major generic-drug companies are producing drugs that are at least equivalent, and in some cases, even better.

"The reality is that there haven't been complaints because of treatment failure," says pharmacist Madeline Feinberg, director of the Elder-Health Program, a consumer drug-education program for older people and care-givers at the University of Maryland's School of Pharmacy. "To my knowledge, no legal cases have established a problem or a difference in the effectiveness between approved generics and brand name drugs in any court of law. When a generic product has been approved by the FDA as bioequivalent, this means that it will behave the same in the body.

"If a patient starting a new medication is advised by his doctor or pharmacist to use a generic," she says, "the patient should be comfortable with that recommendation, and take advantage of the cost savings."

On the other hand, Ms. Feinberg points out, some drugs are not available generically because they are protected by patent, or they're simply not produced because there's not a large demand for that medication. Other generics are available, but are not bioequivalent. These generics can *not* be substituted for the brand name drug because they don't behave the same way in the body. For example, the generic of the drug Dilantin (phenytoin) behaves differently in the body and should not be substituted without physician approval. "If you were on Lanoxin and you wanted a generic," says Ms. Feinberg, "I would discourage it because this is a very potent drug and I would not want to bring in any more variability. Besides that, Lanoxin is relatively inexpensive, and cost savings would be insignificant."

According to many pharmacists, it's not advisable for elderly people who are being successfully maintained on several different medications to switch brands. "For people with multiple diseases, who may be frail and debilitated, it's important to introduce as little change as possible," says Ms. Feinberg. "They should probably keep their drug regimen consistent. The margin of safety for elderly people is narrower, and they should reduce any chances for trouble by staying with the same manufacturer, whether it's a brand or generic drug, regardless of the savings. It's not worth it. They have enough changes going on in their bodies as it is! They can't afford to be exposed to any more change."

Another reason older people taking more than one

medicine might not switch to a generic drug from a brand they're used to is that the generic drug product may often *look* different from the original drug. It can be a different color or a different shape, which can be very confusing for people who identify the drug by the way it looks, not by the label.

"If they ever do get a drug that looks different, they should ask about it," says Ms. Feinberg. "They might assume it's a generic when it's not. For all they know, it could be someone else's medicine that they got by mistake. They need to read the label to know what they're getting.

"It's also important, if they're getting a generic drug, that they ask the pharmacist to put the brand name of the drug in parentheses *after* the generic name on the label. For instance, some pharmacies will put 'propranolol (substitute for Inderal)' on the label, but other pharmacies don't do that automatically. If the customer has one bottle of pills that says propranolol and another, with different-looking pills, that says Inderal, he might think he is taking two different medications, when in fact he's taking a double dose of the exact same thing!"

GENERIC DRUGS*

- DO ask your doctor if there's a generic equivalent for your medication.
- DON'T change dosage forms without asking your doctor. For instance, if you're changing from a brand name drug to a generic drug, don't change drug forms. Don't, for instance, change from a tablet to a liquid—even if the substance is the same—without consulting your doctor or pharmacist first.

---

*Reprinted with permission from the Parke-Davis Center for the Ed-

> - DON'T change dosage forms when you get a refill. Get exactly what you had before unless your pharmacist or doctor has given you the green light on it.
> - DO make sure you inform your doctor and your pharmacist if you make any changes in when or how much of the medication you're taking.

Quality Products

Most independent drugstores and chain drugstores usually have good quality control of their products and can be counted on to have reputable products.

Buying your drugs through the mail is more risky. Mail-order drugs are very price-oriented. Some mail-order businesses are reliable, but it's very difficult to know whether they have consistent quality-control standards. One pharmacist I spoke with said, "They're the prostitutes of the profession. They jump from bed to bed with buyers and distributors, and their buying policies are motivated by price—not quality—control. You can find a few that are good, but for the most part, they're a lot of bad apples." Another problem with mail-order prescriptions is that they eliminate the supervisory role of the pharmacist.

One mail-order pharmacy business that is considered exceptionally good, however, is the AARP Pharmacy Service in Alexandria, Virginia, which is part of the American Association of Retired Persons. This service, which has been in operation for a number of years, delivers prescriptions and health care products postage paid within a few days' time of receiving the prescrip-

ucation of the Elderly, and Elder-Health Program, University of Maryland School of Pharmacy, Baltimore, Md. 21201.

tion. The AARP Pharmacy Service also sends out
medical-information leaflets on medications available
through their service.

YOUR PILL-TAKING REGIMEN

Establishing a routine with your medications can be a
challenge. It's not unlikely that you'll have instructions
to take one pill two times a day (BID), another one
every six hours (QID), and another one after each meal
(pc).

If the doctor, a physician's assistant, nurse, or pharmacist doesn't sit down and help you figure out a pill-
taking regime, you can become very confused and run
into difficulties.

Ask one doctor, nurse, social worker, or phar-
acist to help coordinate your daily regimen of medications. As Caroline Robb says in her recent book,
*The Caregiver's Guide: Helping Older Relatives and
Friends with Health and Safety*, it's essential to have a
commander in chief of medications. Even if you've
worked out a good system for yourself, go over it with
that person. This way there's at least one person besides you who's aware of all the substances going into
your system. It's comforting to know that if for any
reason you lose your mental powers because of a
drug reaction—let's say you begin hallucinating or
talking about someone trying to steal your gold—
someone else may be able to blow the whistle on
what combination of drugs is causing such bizarre
behavior.

Coordination of your medicines is *very* important.

If you have a friend or parent who has poor eyesight or is experiencing mental confusion, help him
(or make sure someone else does) once a week
by sorting out his medicines and putting them into

a pillbox or carton with compartments. Mark the compartments clearly in large, bold letters so that they say, ''Monday morning, Monday noon, Monday evening,'' and so on. Your pharmacist may have a chart, calendar, or pillbox to help you set up such a system.

A chart is also most helpful for people of any age who are taking multiple medications. Anyone who's ever had to take medicines knows that blank moment when you wonder: Did I remember or forget to take my pills at lunchtime? A box with compartments shows you the answer. If the lunch section is empty, you must have already taken those pills! (See chapter 13 for more information on how to manage your medications.)

Always Follow Up
If you take the prescription and you don't feel normal, make sure to call your doctor or pharmacist immediately to tell him about it. If you've done your homework, you'll know which side effects are normal and which ones require a call.

When ''Sonja Miller'' started taking an antibiotic her doctor gave her, she got severe stomach cramps. Instead of calling her doctor, she just discontinued the medication.

''I didn't want to hurt his feelings,'' the seventy-five-year-old librarian said. ''I figured I was feeling better anyway. And I sure felt better after I stopped taking those darn pills!''

Don't worry about hurting your doctor's feelings or making him angry. First of all, he won't be angry—you are simply reporting your reaction to the drug. Even if he does feel badly about what he prescribed, it's still much more important that he know the facts. Without them, he can't do his job well; he can't contribute properly to your health care.

Sometimes, too, by making a call, you can find out

why you're having the reaction. If Ms. Miller had called her doctor, for instance, he probably would have told her that antibiotics are sometimes hard on the stomach, so she should take a cracker along with her pill. Although antibiotics are most effective on an empty stomach, they often cause cramps or nausea, so you might need to eat a little something at the same time you take the medication. As it was, Ms. Miller did not get rid of the walking pneumonia she had been carrying around in her system. Two months later, she was sick again and had to take her antibiotics flat on her back.

Medicine at its best is part of an open communication and interaction between doctor and patient. If you hold up your end of the communication, you'll maximize the benefits of the medicines you use and minimize the risks.

CHAPTER 5

Causes and Effects of Aging—A Path into the Future

"How old would you be if you didn't know how old you was?"

—SATCHEL PAIGE

If you look around you, you'll see tremendous diversity in the energy, interests, and health of people as they age. For many older people, chronological age seems irrelevant. There's the seventy-six-year-old grandmother who's running the New York City Marathon with her son and grandson, and the keen-witted New Jersey doctor who's still practicing medicine every day at the age of one hundred. There are the famous examples of Marc Chagall, Pablo Picasso, P. G. Wodehouse, Winston Churchill, and Somerset Maugham, to name a few, who worked well into their nineties with vigor and imagination. It's easy to find evidence that chronological age renders no magical limits in terms of creativity, judgment, ability, or dexterity.

The other day when I was sitting on my front steps, I waved to a seventy-six-year-old neighbor who was riding her bike home from a tennis game. It struck me suddenly that while she was out slamming the ball back over the net, probably at least one of her former classmates was having trouble lifting her spoon to her mouth.

I also thought of my gym teacher, Rose Kolberg, who at eighty-five still teaches dance exercise classes seven days a week. At five foot six, with soft red hair that complements her sculptured face, Rose still looks lithe and graceful when she moves out from behind her grand

113

piano to show her pupils how to follow through on a
swing stretch to the left.

Although Rose maintains a schedule that would wear
out most forty-year-olds, she finds that her body continues to change in a variety of ways she doesn't like.
"Getting old is no fun," she says. "Don't let anybody
fool you. Old is terrible! I hate it! Everything breaks
down. If it's not one thing, it's another. I know that
even though an infection in my finger gets better, next
week I'll get shingles or something else will go out. I
keep being forced to adjust to it! Last week I moved
my friend's furniture and I hurt my back! Isn't that stupid?! Now they say I shouldn't be moving furniture!"

Although Rose's continuing beauty and verve inspire
her friends and students, she's personally very con-
scious of the ways she's aging within her own body. Her
skin may look like the skin of a much younger woman,
she concedes, and it might be astonishing to others that
she has no wrinkles around her neck. But, she points
out, you should have seen that hip joint that was replaced last summer. Now *that* hip joint was just as old
as it looked! And the same goes for the joints in the
fingers of her left hand—which are getting stiffer, no
matter how much she accompanies her students on the
piano, no matter what kind of gloves she wears to keep
her hands warm, no matter what she eats or what kind
of creams she uses. Doctors have recently found that
she has a rare condition of having too much blood in
her body, so every six weeks, she has to have blood
taken to keep the volume properly balanced.

As Rose Kolberg so aptly demonstrates, experience
with aging varies dramatically from one person to another, but it also varies dramatically within the person's
own body. Now gerontologists can determine our *biological* age by a series of tests that measure our cardiac
function, hearing, lung function, reflexes, and memory.
They're beginning to show us that our bodies age with
as many unpredictable and individual quirks as do our

personalities. Just as a man in his late seventies can sometimes be in much better physical shape than a fifty-five-year-old colleague, various systems within his body can have different levels of health and rates of aging. Age-related changes in one organ don't necessarily predict equivalent changes in other organs.

Let's take a look at Loretta Campbell, for instance. At eighty years of age, Loretta walks three to five miles a day. Her doctor says she seems to have the legs and lungs of a fifty-year-old, but lately her kidneys have been behaving as if they were eighty-five or ninety years old. The skin on Loretta's face is smooth and rosy, like the skin of a sixty-year-old, and yet she has purple-blue veins that stand out on her hands and make them look ancient.

"We do know that the changes in different organs are variable," says Dr. J. Edwin Seegmiller, director of the Institute for Research on Aging at the University of California at San Diego's School of Medicine. "We also know that the older people become, the less like each other they become. There's a much larger difference between people physiologically at the age of seventy than there is at forty. We've also learned that if we understand how fast your kidney is aging, that does *not* help us understand how your heart is aging."

EXPLORING THE MYSTERIES OF AGING

Like our knowledge of aging, geriatric research is relatively new. In the past ten years, however, it has made enormous advances. The National Institute of Aging (NIA) was established in 1976 under the National Institutes of Health in Bethesda, Maryland, with the promising mandate to pursue research into the biological, medical, social, and behavioral aspects of the process of aging. While the NIA's budget has been much smaller than many other medical research budgets, the issues the NIA addresses could ultimately save taxpayers billions of dollars. Some researchers project that in the year 2000, an increased number of older people will need nearly three times the hospital care they required in 1980 and that we'll be spending more than $200 billion a year on health care for them if we continue in our present patterns. Obviously, real answers to how people can stay healthy longer would be more than cost-effective.

In 1991, Congress agreed to raise the NIA's budget to $323.8 million. Overall, the total federal budget designated for aging research is $548.3 million—money that will be put to good use in unraveling the mysteries of aging and finding the answers to real-life issues that face our older population. If research on aging and age-related diseases led to finding a cause and treatment for only one disease, such as Alzheimer's, the national savings in health-care costs alone would be phenomenal. But certainly, the answers still elude us when it comes to the fundamental questions of what causes aging and how we can slow down its process to extend our lives.

Dr. Tom Nicholson, astronomer and director of the Museum of Natural History in New York City, likens the mystery of aging to the mystery of the stars. "Longevity is a far more complex problem than it was ever seen to be," Dr. Nicholson told a group of scientists and doctors gathered in New York in the spring of 1986 for a conference on the biological aspects of aging. "It reminds me of the story of Einstein asking a student how he thought a star worked. The student said, 'Oh, I don't know. It looks pretty simple.' Einstein said, 'If you were a hundred thousand light-years away, you'd look pretty simple, too.' Eventually we'll be able to unscramble our understanding of aging and longevity, just as we've unscrambled our understanding of stars."

We have a sense, for instance, that our age can't be measured purely by chronology, but is dramatically influenced by the specter of our attitudes, our activities, and our health. Dr. Nicolson pointed out that in a similar way, the age of stars isn't measured by chronological age, but has to do with metabolism and maturity. Their *specter* has to do with temperature and *spectral* classifications.

We still have a lot to learn about longevity. Just *why* we age may be due to extrinsic factors in the environment that produce changes in the human organism—or it may also be intrinsic, in other words, the result of changes, some of which also may be triggered by the environment—that are internal and predetermined. Are we affected more by our life-style and what we take into our bodies, or by the genes we inherited from our parents? How do our life-styles interact with our genes?

SOME REASONABLE HYPOTHESES

At this time, scientists have many plausible theories about the causes of aging, some considered more likely than others. Dr. Edward Schneider, former deputy director of the National Institute of Aging, who is now dean of the Andrus Gerontology Center at the University of Southern California, says there are at least twenty-five or thirty hypotheses. The complexity of the aging process is attested to by the large number of hypotheses being considered.

One theory suggests that ordinary wear and tear causes our bodies to "give out" due to harmful substances we breathe and eat or to natural processes within the body that "give out" due to the stresses of being alive. The "wear and tear" theory may apply to different levels of body organisms, from a degeneration of the joints of a runner down to a subcellular level for the accumulation of pigments.

Another intriguing theory suggests that we have biological clocks built into our genetic programs. These clocks are set when we're born and they tick away—

within either all or (more likely) some of our cells—
and determine when we mature, when we age, and when
we die. An example of the "cell pacemaker" that's most
established is the loss of egg cells from the ovary. Why
women have a fixed number of cells that are progressively lost until menopause is still poorly understood,
but may lead us to an understanding of how the programs of our own life expectancy are computed.

A long-standing hypothesis that's now being given
critical testing with modern techniques is that the DNA,
the machinery in every cell body, may cause malfunc-
tion in the cells that leads to aging. While certain aspects of this DNA-mutation or "error" theory have
been laid to rest, the mutation theory still holds interest
and remains a highly speculative and open question.

A newer and promising research area concerns the
many hormonal changes that occur across the human
lifespan. The most dramatic of these changes occurs at
menopause, when the steroids of the ovaries virtually
disappear with ovarian exhaustion, leading to major deficits of estrogen and progesterone. However, there are
other changes that occur in mid-life and later in both
sexes, such as altered regulation of insulin and growth
hormone. In addition, there's another steroid referred
to as DHEA-S, which begins to change before mid-life
in healthy adults and declines to very low values after
seventy and eighty years of age. The significance of the
change isn't known, but DHEA-S has interesting and
provocative properties: when given to laboratory mice,
it seems to retard carcinogenesis and prevent obesity.
It therefore may have a role in some of the aspects of
increased cancer with age. Although this is an extremely speculative hypothesis, steroids may be found
to play a significant role in the breakdowns involved in
aging.

Previous understanding of how we age indicated that
we experience major impairments of the immune system as we grow older, but these may be much less than

they were assumed to be. There's great uncertainty at this point about impaired immunological responses. Some of the hormones produced by the thymus gland that regulate the immunological function seem to be sharply decreased during aging, but the functional consequences are not fully understood.

While absolute answers still evade us, great progress has been made, through the use of modern techniques, in testing these and many other reasonable hypotheses. Certainly, while there's more hope for understanding the complex mysteries involved in aging, there's less optimism among scientists about finding one single theory that will explain all aspects of aging. The expectation is that aging will be understood as many different processes with different mechanisms that can be traced in some cases to earliest development and that occur across the entire life span, from conception until old age.

"Aging is multicausal," says Dr. Schneider. "Ten years ago we heard arguments that cancer could be explained by only one cause, but now we know that even cancer is multicausal. It's encouraging to hear agreement among scientists that aging has many causes on many levels—molecular, cellular, environmental."

The prospect of scientific breakthroughs that give us an understanding of the root causes of aging holds great promise for tomorrow's older people. As Dr. Robert Butler points out, a real interweaving of this science with improved health has the potential to leapfrog us once again into further life extensions and increased life expectancy.

"It was not an understanding of the biology of aging that led us to the longevity revolution," says Dr. Butler. "Imagine what we might do *with* an understanding of it!"

Some day we may have longevity pills we can pop to repair chinks in the armor of our DNA, reset the aging-clocks in our cells, or protect our systems from the dangers in our environment. Perhaps we'll be able to add years to our life spans. Until then, however, we'll continue to live day-to-day with the basic biology of aging.

OUR BASIC BIOLOGY

When I try to understand how the body functions as it ages, I envision each person as a large, detailed map. It's as if all of us have interconnecting communities living within one large metropolitan area that makes up our bodies. All of these communities may have been established at approximately the same point in time, but their development and varying rates of activity, change, population growth, crisis, and decline have influenced them in different ways. Some of the communities can still be considered young and thriving, others remain fairly stable, and still others are on the decline.

All that activity is taking place within the body—the greater metropolitan area. To keep the entire area running smoothly, each community's acute problems must be addressed as they occur. For instance, if major thoroughfares get blocked, they must be reopened. Sometimes certain traffic lights go out; detours must be established, and the traffic must be redirected. The tremendous range both within one individual's body and from one person to the next is the basis for saying that we become more heterogeneous, as opposed to homogeneous, as we age.

What an idiosyncratic process it is! Physiologically things happen to us at highly differing rates. Just because your friend is the same age you are doesn't mean you'll be experiencing the same things.

SIGNS OF AGING

On the other hand, there are some universals. Even though they come at different times and at different rates, older people share many telltale signs of aging. Even before you experience any loss in your vision or hearing, you may notice changes in your skin. It will probably be less moist and less resilient. It may become leathery and may get aging spots or patches of dryness. Although we've learned that staying out of the sun and not smoking keeps skin younger-looking, wrinkled skin remains a hallmark of aging.

One day it may seem that you have gotten shorter. If this happens, it is probably due to a change in your skeletal system. A statural decline, a loss of height or a change in posture, is due primarily to a loss of height when the vertebral column shortens. Bone changes occur primarily because of decreased mineral content. Not all people experience a loss of physical stature, but depending on your lifetime diet, how much calcium you've had, and other factors, there may be a change in how strong your bones are. They may be more brittle and curved. If you don't stand as straight as you used to, it may be that you are off balance because your center of gravity has shifted.

Another factor that can create a different perception of your balance is a change in proprioception. This is knowing where your body is in relation to your surroundings. Some people, no matter what age they are, bump into tables and doors and even walls. If this didn't happen to you when you were younger, count your blessings. If it starts happening to you when you're older, talk to your doctor about it, but also try to arrange your furniture so that you have clear paths and easy movement around your home. Some older people also have decreased reflex time, so they can't dodge something that's falling toward them or sidestep a slippery spot as quickly as they once might have.

Besides your hair changing color and texture and a thinning of the rest of your body hair, your fingernails and toenails may become thicker, harder, and more brittle.

These external changes are connected to changes that are going on *inside* your body—changes within your cells, organs, and organ systems. This includes changes in enzymes, hormones, and tissues, which affect all your body functions. No one definitively knows *why* these changes occur, but they do. Internal changes, progressing at various rates, have effects we can feel on occasion but cannot see. Sometimes we can't feel them either. We can't see the tissues that support a lot of our organs, but they may be becoming thicker and it may become more difficult for nutrients and oxygen to be exchanged. For example, the little sacks on the external part of the lungs—the alveoli—are not as resilient as they once were. They're thicker, so there can be less exchange of carbon dioxide and oxygen than there used to be.

Although it's believed that physical decline associated with aging can eventually be postponed if not reversed, aging does impose some biological limits. In the cardiovascular system, veins, capillaries, and arteries lose elasticity and tend to become less pliant. The heart decreases its output, and there's often an increase in the resistance to blood flow because of a narrowing of blood vessels due to disease. When this happens, certain vital organs don't have the same flow of blood through them as they used to. When blood flow to the brain and the kidney is decreased because of this natural process, these highly vascular organs are affected.

In addition to some natural weakening of the capacity of the heart and lungs, metabolism and reflexes slow down as well. The central nervous system often processes information less rapidly than it once did, and often slows down reaction time. And although there is growing hope that the immune system can be kept young, evidence from research is strong that the immune system does decline. Whether this decline results from diet and life-style or genetic inheritance, or both, the result is that resistance to infections and certain diseases is usually lowered with age, and it takes longer to recover from certain injuries and illnesses.

Of course any of the changes that take place in your body are not simultaneous or entirely predictable. As we've said, biological aging is a highly individual process.

BODY SIGNALS CHANGE

The physiological changes occurring as you age often make it much more difficult to diagnose diseases. The changes in your system mean that when you get an illness, you don't necessarily have the classic symptoms of that disease that you would have had when you were younger.

When seventy-three-year-old Charlie Sampson went to see his doctor for his six-month checkup, he didn't have a high fever or bad cough. But Charlie's doctor, alert to changes in Charlie's demeanor, noticed that Charlie didn't look well. He was slightly pale and didn't seem to be as ebullient as usual. When he inquired, he found that Charlie hadn't been feeling well. He was tired, but fatigue was his only identifiable "symptom." His doctor ordered a chest X ray and discovered that Charlie had pneumonia.

Because symptoms aren't predictable and because the disease manifestations are more idiosyncratic and more difficult to find, physicians treating older people have to have a higher degree of suspicion about any changes in the patient. For example, an older person can have a "silent heart attack" that has no outer manifestations. An older person who has a fever or an infected toe may also indicate it by a change in mental demeanor and status—not with chills, a flushed, hot face, or profuse sweating. Whereas a younger person with a ruptured appendix would probably be cramping, vomiting, and feeling as if he were going to die, an older person in the same critical condition might only have a sore throat or a high fever, with no cramps or nausea at all.

That symptoms are different in older people than they are in younger people probably has to do with the fact that they have less reserve in the body, says Dr. Michael Freedman at New York University Medical Center. "The classic symptom is where you don't develop a fever as quickly, so you don't release the things that give you fever as quickly," he says. "With the differences in indications of pain, it probably has to do with differences in nerve conduction. If you think about it, the classic descriptions of disease came from describing the symptoms of younger people. But if we had described older patients first, younger people would be the ones with the odd symptoms. Older people are the ones who get more of these diseases, so actually, the classic descriptions are the ones that are atypical!"

Dr. Charles Herrera, who was acting chief of the Coffey Geriatrics Clinic at Mount Sinai Hospital when I interviewed him, said that when you're dealing with older people, your index of suspicion has to operate at a higher degree. "You have to ask questions in a way that you can get answers," he says. "What's important to watch for is *change* of any kind. What's important in geriatric medicine is your interest in the whole person with whom you're dealing. You have to be alert to details and to differences within the same person."

Reactions Are Different
Clearly, when you're older, your body isn't the same as it was before. What are the implications of these differences? What can you expect? What changes will you see in how your body deals with food and medicine when you are fifty, sixty, seventy, eighty, ninety, one hundred, and one hundred and ten?

In terms of the body's ability to process medicines, foods, and other things you put into your system, you will probably notice a progression of subtle changes. You may notice that you react differently to various substances, such as alcohol, cigarette smoke, and certain foods, than you did when you were younger. It might be, for instance, that red wine will start giving you headaches, or a particular food you used to love will make you feel slightly nauseated. At some point, food simply may taste different than it used to. In most people, the sense of smell declines after age sixty-five. Your taste buds change, too, so you may need to use various herbs and spices to make food taste more appealing. Although some of these changes may be unpleasant, they shouldn't be a source of pain or sickness. Subtle changes require subtle adaptations. When it comes to the way your body reacts to medications as you age, however, the differences can be of monumental importance. And although the aging of your various internal systems is unseen, it can have dramatic effects on the normal routine of taking medicine.

The way your body responds to a medicine depends on a vast number of factors. "As people get older, they become prone to declines at highly differing rates," says Dr. William Gershell, a geriatric psychiatrist and assistant clinical professor of psychiatry at the Mount Sinai School of Medicine. "How their bodies handle medications they are given depends on their rates of aging, their differing degrees of health, and the number of physical conditions and associated conditions that are being treated—along with an individual's emotional reactions to those conditions that affect their overall functioning." If we go back to our analogy of the greater metropolitan area, we can compare the way medicine goes through the body to the way that traffic flows through densely populated communities that have construction underway at various sites. There are some detours, some narrowing of streets, some rather large potholes to avoid, some traffic signals that are simply out of commission, and sometimes a few conflicts raging here or there that may or may not get addressed or resolved.

Some common factors that can affect the way your body handles a particular medicine or medicines include the way the drug is absorbed, distributed, metabolized, excreted, and received at the site for which it's intended. Depending on how quickly you digest your food and eliminate it, you keep it in your body for longer or shorter periods of time. The same goes for your medicines.

A CHANGING LANDSCAPE

When you take a medicine, it must be absorbed by the gastrointestinal tract before it enters the bloodstream to be carried to its site of action. As you age, your intestinal blood flow is decreased, as are the number of absorbing cells and therefore the absorbing surface. As your body ages, the amount of water in it decreases, and this also affects the way the drug is absorbed. All of these effects may result in a delay or a reduction of the way the drug is absorbed. If the acid secretion in your stomach is impaired, it may compound the problem by altering the solubility of some drugs.

As your body gets older, there's usually a decrease in lean body mass and muscle and an increase in fat. This changes the amount and concentration of specific drugs in the bloodstream and in the tissues. Many psychotropic drugs are likely to be fatty-tissue-soluble; these medicines can be distributed more widely and tend to have a longer stay than they would if there weren't as much fat.

The way medicines are metabolized—changed physically and chemically—also changes in the aging body. When medicines are absorbed into your body, they eventually reach the liver, which is the major detoxifying organ in the body. The liver's job is to take out the poisons and purify the substance. The mechanism by which the body converts the medicines into compounds that can be used by the body is termed biotransformation. Although this process can occur in other organs, it primarily occurs in the liver.

The biotransformation of drugs generally occurs more slowly with age. Age-related changes in the size of the liver, the structure of the tissue, and the blood flow are thought to be changes that contribute to this effect.

Difficulties with the Filtration System

Further complicating matters is the rate at which medicines are excreted. The kidney is our major filtration system, and if it's not functioning effectively, more of the drug will remain in the system. For many older people, the kidney function slows down. Some studies say that by the time a person is seventy or eighty years old, his kidney function has decreased by 50 percent. Also, in many people the rate of the concentration of substances excreted from the body decreases considerably after the age of seventy.

When drugs leave the body at a slower rate, this means that they stay longer in the body, which increases the likelihood that a person will build up a larger supply of any particular drug than might be assumed from the dosage he's taking. This is a major reason that doctors start older patients on smaller drug doses instead of "normal" adult doses. According to some recent studies, however, a significant minority of older people have no change in their kidneys as they grow older. The rate of their excretion remains constant, as does the concentration of substances excreted. In these patients, reducing the medication can result in undermedication.

Many older people are smaller in height and weight when compared with today's younger people. This may be one of the reasons that normal drug doses (FDA standard doses) are usually too high for many older people to handle.

Additionally, instead of going where it's supposed to go, medicine may be circulating more freely in an older body in greater concentrations. That happens when there's a decrease in the ability of the body to bind the various components of drugs. Many drugs bind, in particular, to a protein called albumin, which is in the liquid part of our blood. As we get older, we may have less albumin in our bodies.

When drugs are not in a bound form within the body, they're potentially more toxic. An example of one drug displacing another from a binding site and causing a toxic effect is when a person of any age takes aspirin along with Coumadin, which is prescribed for problems with too much blood clotting. The Coumadin exists in two forms, bound and unbound. When aspirin is taken, it displaces the Coumadin bound to the albumin and causes there to be too much free Coumadin in the body. In extreme cases, this can cause the patient to bleed to death.

The accumulation of unbound drugs can also cause an increase or decrease in sensitivity in places like the heart, the spleen, or the blood, where the action is located. The drugs in your body compete for receptor sites on these organs, and reduced plasma protein in the blood intensifies the competition among drugs for binding sites. Just as land developers compete for territory, so, too, drugs compete for choice spots in your body. It's an ongoing competition. One may have claim of the territory for a certain period of time and then get taken over or pushed out by another medicine that's more of a bully.

Problems caused by reductions in binding in the elderly have been found in Dilantin (which is taken for seizures), Coumadin, Demerol (a narcotic painkiller), and heparin, an anticoagulant.

When a doctor is giving you a chosen medicine, his

goal is to maintain a proper concentration. If a constant and stable amount of the drug can be maintained, the balanced effect that you and your doctor want is achieved. But when the drug isn't absorbed as well as usual, distributed as rapidly, metabolized as thoroughly, or excreted at "normal" rates—in other words, at younger rates—then it's often difficult to establish and maintain the proper dosage.

If you're older, remember that the "standard dose" is based on what younger patients need, and it may very likely be too much for you.

"When it comes to being old and using medicines, think little," says my 105-pound, five-foot-tall aunt who's a former nurse. "That's easy for me to say because I'm little, but the same rule should apply to most older people, even to the big guys."

CHAPTER 6

How Your Body Responds to Drugs— Side Effects, Allergic Reactions, and Toxic Reactions

> "Alice had not a moment to think about stopping herself before she found herself falling down a very deep well. . . . Down, down, down. Would the fall *never* come to an end!
>
> " 'What a curious feeling!' said Alice. 'I must be shutting up like a telescope.' And so it was indeed: she was now only ten inches high."
>
> —LEWIS CARROLL
> *Alice's Adventures in Wonderland*

"There's no such thing as a drug without side effects," says Dr. Bernard Mehl, director of the Department of Pharmacy at Mount Sinai Medical Center in New York City. "It's just a matter of how serious they are and how often they happen."

The way Alice felt as she was falling down the rabbit hole—or later when she drank the poison and got smaller while the world around her got bigger—is not entirely unlike the side effects Helen Ahern experienced after she was put on nadolol (Corgard) for hypertension.

"At first I began to feel real depressed," says seventy-seven-year-old Helen Ahern, a nurse, schoolteacher, mother of five, and grandmother of eleven, who lives in New Hartford, Connecticut, with her husband.

"I'm not used to being depressed, and I felt like something was really wrong, but I couldn't think what was wrong. Everything seemed awful. I was worried about a lot of things, but I felt hopeless. Whatever it was, I knew I couldn't do anything about it. I couldn't even think about eating anything. Even food seemed terrible to me.

"It took over my life. I was turning in on myself, like I was getting smaller and smaller and I wanted to withdraw from the human race.

"I just went to bed. I didn't have it in me to do anything about the way I felt. Fortunately, our daughter-in-law Kathy, who's a nurse, was visiting us, and she got on the phone and called my doctor. She told him something was really wrong with me and asked him if it could be my medicines. It had never occurred to me that it might be my medicines.

"He suggested that I stop taking whatever I was taking and see if I felt better. I stopped everything, and within a day or two, I was better. I started feeling normal again, and then it was like a bad dream. I went in to see him, and he took me off Corgard for good. He wanted me on something to control my blood pressure, because it had been shooting up. I suggested that whatever he decided to give me, he start me on a quarter of a tablet instead of full strength. He started me on Tenormin—and told me to break it in half and then break it in half again. It wasn't so hard on me, even at the beginning. He gradually increased it to one-half tablet. Now my blood pressure is controlled with one-half tablet of Tenormin and a diuretic, and it's been very helpful."

When you're talking about reactions to medications, you're talking about a range—minor to severe—of physical and emotional responses.

"Side effects" are harmful. They are what can happen to you *in addition* to what the drug is supposed to do for you. In *The Nurse's Guide to Drugs*, side effects are described as "any drug effect that's other than the therapeutically intended effect." If, for instance, the intended therapeutic effect of a medicine is to lower your blood pressure and it does that and *also* makes you depressed or it makes you urinate a lot, then you're experiencing a side effect of the drug. You may be having a common physical side effect if you experience either constipation or diarrhea, headaches, dry mouth, blurred vision, nausea, dizziness, loss of hearing, sensitivity to light, ringing in your ears, loss of bladder control, urinary retention, tiredness, drowsiness, or lethargy. It used to be that medicines didn't work very well and that their side effects far outweighed their benefits. Now the effectiveness of medicines is so much greater than it used to be that we're willing to take the medicines and put up with expected side effects. Not everyone experiences the side effects of a particular drug in the same way, however. Some people don't experience any side effects, whereas for others, the effect of the drug on their systems produces dramatic reactions. For Helen, the side effects far outweighed the benefits.

"Any medicine is a double-edged sword," says Dr. William Gershell at the Mount Sinai School of Medicine. "Medicine has the capacity to help us if it's presented in a suitable and appropriate way. That capacity to help is balanced against its capacity to create side effects that may add to your problem or complicate it."

Some direct chemical effects, not considered side effects because they're not harmful, are to be expected and are benign and unavoidable. For instance, if you have a urinary infection and you take Pyridium to ease the pain for it, along with your antibiotic, your urine will turn red-orange because Pyridium is a dye. Sometimes when people haven't been warned about this predictable effect, which is not at all harmful, they think they're bleeding or that the infection is getting worse. As a result, they sometimes stop the medication and they're more uncomfortable than necessary during their healing process.

Some common side effects to medications can seem minor, but according to *Pharmacy Practice for the Geriatric Patient*, even a side effect such as dryness of the mouth can be troublesome and harmful in elderly patients. When a person has a persistently dry mouth, for instance, it can make the use of dentures difficult and cause dental complications. Additionally, chewing and swallowing become more difficult and can contribute to problems of malnutrition in older individuals. The same is true of drugs that make you lose your sense of taste or make you too lethargic to eat.

Just as a dry mouth can lead to serious complications, greatly reduced or increased appetite can also be a real problem. In treating depression, antidepressants are often prescribed to increase the appetite of depressed people. In one study of elderly patients placed on tricyclic antidepressant medicine, however, more than a third had excessive appetites resulting from their drug treatment. Thirty-four percent said they were craving sweet foods and that cravings tended to be most pronounced in the evenings. These appetite changes were correlated with weight gain and with higher doses of the antidepressant, but there wasn't any correlation with alleviation from depression.

Sometimes, a particular medicine combined with your particular personality will make you feel peculiar. A medicine that speeds you up when you are used to a slow and steady pace, for instance, can make you feel slightly frantic. The reverse is also true. These are called "psychotropic" drug effects. If you're normally low-key and a medicine such as an amphetamine speeds you up, it can create anxiety or a heightened sense of apprehensiveness. Some other psychotropic side effects from the medicine you're taking may include nervousness, agitation, depression, euphoria, and excitement. When a medicine you're taking alters your mood or the way you feel, you'll want to work with your doctor to make the necessary adjustments.

SIDE EFFECTS: A HOST OF POSSIBILITIES

Sometimes a side effect in an older person makes it difficult to distinguish between the symptoms of the condition being treated and the effects of the drug or symptoms of a supposedly new condition.

When eighty-five-year-old Rose Anderson was having a great deal of pain in her feet from arthritis, for example, she wasn't getting very much sleep at night. She was tired and groggy during the day, which everyone assumed was from not sleeping at night. One day when her sister visited, however, she found Rose "very despondent" and groggy and wondered if perhaps she'd had another stroke. Rose, who is normally quite enthusiastic, said she didn't care if she lived or died. Knowing that Rose is "never like that," her sister correctly suspected that medication was causing Rose's lethargy, not her lack of sleep. She found out that Rose's doctor had put her on two tablets of a salicylate per day because of the pain she was having in her feet. One time when she was in a great deal of pain, she had called the doctor's vacation stand-in, who told her to take four salicylate tablets a day instead of two. She did this for several days and became more and more depressed and confused. She was relieved at having no pain, but by then her speech was slurred and she couldn't think. When her doctor returned from vacation, he had her discontinue the medicine altogether. Within a day and a half, she'd improved remarkably.

Some side effects can change your total demeanor, leading others to think that you're failing rapidly or that you've acquired a new disease. This often happens when behavior caused by medication makes you confused and disoriented, leading others to think that you're becoming demented or "senile." You may start forgetting what you were saying in the middle of a sentence, wondering which way to turn when you're walking what was once a familiar route. You may be too mixed up to remember that your medicine could be causing this behavior. Make sure to let your friends or children know ahead of time that confusion is sometimes a symptom of a drug reaction. Tell them that if you ever start acting "funny," they should check with your doctor about the possibility of your having a response to a medication. If a parent or friend sixty-five or over suddenly starts forgetting things, is absentminded, confused about behavior, and has speech or hearing problems, he or she may be suffering from drug reactions. Check immediately with the person's doctor about medications.

Check Medications First

Sometimes physicians misread a patient's drug reactions. If they believe that they're seeing a new disease manifestation, they often order expensive tests or do exploratory surgery to find out what's wrong—or corrective surgery to correct the condition. This also happens when a patient who develops new "symptoms" goes to a different doctor to treat the problem instead of going back to the same doctor. Patients who go from one doctor to the next also often fail to tell the doctor what medications they're taking, and the new doctor can add to the complications by prescribing medications she thinks are addressing a specific disease, when all that is actually needed is to stop or change the medication causing the reactions.

Unfortunately, even when a patient stays with the same doctor, the doctor sometimes overlooks the possibility of drug reactions and thinks he's seeing a new and separate condition. This happened to Faith Smiley when she had a hysterectomy that should have been fairly routine. By the third or fourth day after surgery, however, she wasn't able to keep any food down or to get out of bed. She was dehydrated, and when she ate anything, she threw it up. She couldn't even take a sip of water. Every day she got sicker and sicker. Faith's doctor thought she might have a blockage and told her husband that he might have to do exploratory surgery.

"I'd told my doctor ahead of time that I'd gotten very sick before from taking Demerol," says Faith. "Demerol is like codeine and makes me deathly sick, but since I'd told him about it, I never suspected I was on it. I got too sick, frankly, to even be able to think. I started feeling as if I was going to die and there wasn't anything I could do about it." Faith was in critical condition when her sister visited and suddenly had the impulse to ask the doctor what was in the bottle that was being fed to Faith intravenously. When the doctor stopped the Demerol, which was poisoning her, Faith began to get better. Fortunately, she didn't undergo surgery for a nonexistent blockage.

The moral of Faith's story is that you have to be vigilant all the time. Even if you've told your doctor that you're allergic to a medication, even if you've given him a history that includes adverse reactions to certain drugs, find out everything you need to know about the medication you're taking. If you're undergoing treatment for a certain condition, or entering a hospital, tell your family members to be vigilant on your behalf. If anything odd happens to you while you're on a medication, always suspect that medication, and always go back to the same doctor before you begin to take another medication or undergo diagnostic tests or exploratory surgery for a supposedly "new" condition.

The Lesser of Two Evils

Some kind of side effect almost universally occurs in conjunction with the drug consumed. Usually these reactions are tolerated because balancing the therapeutic effect against the side effect offers more comfort than distress. Hay fever sufferers who take chlorpheniramine

(Chlortrimeton), for instance, sometimes find that they get somewhat drowsy on the medication but feel that drowsiness is a small price to pay compared with constant sneezing and stuffiness. Drowsiness is also an expected side effect of Dramamine, but people who take it would rather be a little sleepy than motion-sick. Also, the side effect wears off with time.

Even when the side effect is more severe, we might decide that it's the lesser of two evils. For instance, when ninety-four-year old "Ina Dutton" got slightly confused from her heart medicine, she didn't like it. Nevertheless, given a choice between slight confusion on occasion and staying alive, she preferred staying alive. Her sons, who consulted regularly with her doctor, were also well aware of the trade-offs. When they suggested a lower dosage to the doctor, he tried it, and it lessened Ina's confusion considerably.

Sixty-nine-year-old Dianne West also makes a trade-off with her medicine. She takes a drug called Ameoterone for her heart arrythmias; that drug keeps her alive. Although she's fully aware that the drug may compromise her lung function and her thyroid function, she chooses to take it and accept the possible consequences.

Side Effects from Overdoses

It's not at all unusual for older people to be overdosed. This isn't necessarily due to their own mistakes in taking their medicine. Sometimes the doctor has prescribed too strong a dose. Other times, it's because of the way the body is processing, storing, and eliminating the drug, or because weight fluctuations lead to an overdose. Side effects from overdoses can create harmful conditions and can often be dealt with by the patient's adjusting the dosage or changing medicines.

Anita's mother, in her seventies, was living alone after the death of her husband. She was depressed, but Anita noticed that every time her mother rose from a sitting position, she steadied herself on whatever was near. When she asked her why, her mother said she felt dizzy and light-headed whenever she stood up. She blamed it on depression.

"I just can't get over Ben's death," she said several times. "I know I'll feel better when I get past the first six months." Because Anita is a nurse, and because she knew her mother was taking reserpine for her hypertension, she guessed that her mother might be having a reaction to the reserpine. Anita called her mother's doctor, whose first response was to explain that Anita's mother, his patient, was feeling particularly low because her husband had died.

"I think that's true," Anita said, "but she's been depressed before without being so lethargic. Also, the dizziness and light-headedness don't fit. How about trying to lower the dosage and see what happens?"

The doctor did lower the dosage; the depression lifted, and the light-headedness and dizziness disappeared—these symptoms were directly related to too much reserpine built up in her system.

Your Perfect Dosage

Most side effects are related to the amount of medicine given and the amount of the drug circulating in the body. As we've said before, getting the dosage exactly right for each particular patient is very difficult.

When giving you a medication, doctors are aware of a "therapeutic index," which measures a certain range of plasma concentrations in the body. Most drugs have very specific "therapeutic windows" at which the drug is concentrated enough to be effective, but not so much that it creates side effects. The "windows" of some drugs are very small; it's difficult for those drugs to be effective without side effects. The "windows" on other drugs are large. Some drugs, like penicillin, can be effective even when there is a vast difference between the amount you give and the number of milligrams that are in the blood.

At very low concentrations, a certain drug may not be effective, and yet at high concentrations, negative side effects will occur. It's ideal to have drugs that work at low levels of concentration without side effects. Some drugs have side effects at lower concentrations, but most have side effects at higher levels.

Just as no two thumbprints are exactly alike, no two people react to or tolerate medicines in all the same ways. Many variables can create an overdose or under-dose effect, particularly in an older person. The perfect dose for you might be quite different from someone else's perfect dose because of your weight, sex, age, and the way the drug metabolizes in your system. Other factors to consider can include your physical and emotional state, your recent pattern of use with the same drug and other drugs, how tired you are, and how much of the drug in question has been secreted from your body. When the doctor gives you a new medicine, he's conducting an experiment of sorts—and he has to depend on your compliance and your reports back to him to observe the effects of the prescription. He has to make sure there are no side effects, and he also has to watch to see that the drug is doing what it's supposed to do.

Side Effects That Work to Your Advantage

Occasionally, side effects can be put to good clinical use. In these cases, physicians can sometimes give one medicine to effectively treat the symptoms of two separate conditions. For instance, some drugs that are used for treating Parkinson's disease have the secondary effect of lowering a person's blood pressure. While this drug effect could cause an untoward reaction if it was coupled with another antihypertensive medication, it serves the purpose of cutting down on medications rather than increasing them.

Another drug, Elavil, which is used as an antidepressant, usually causes drowsiness. If a patient also complains of insomnia, the physician can prescribe Elavil and tell the patient to take one larger dose at night before going to bed rather than taking three or four doses during the day. It serves as a sleeping pill and still achieves its goals as an antidepressant.

The Statute of Limitations

Sometimes drugs that may have been useful for a short period of time not only outlive their usefulness, they become downright harmful. Their double-edged nature backfires. If a doctor isn't extremely cautious, and if he doesn't review the use of the patient's ongoing medications, the patient may develop another disease as a result of the medication he's on. Patients who take diuretics over a period of time, for instance, can sometimes develop gout as a result. Another example of this is the blood thinner warfarin (Coumadin), which many heart patients are given. This is an important and useful drug, but if the dosage isn't carefully monitored, the patient can become anemic. At the least, this can develop a need for iron; at the worst, a person can die from internal bleeding. Sometimes situations that result from unmonitored drug use over a long period of time can be dealt with simply by cutting down or cutting out the offending medicine, before things get out of hand, as they did for "Max Wachtell."

Max, a retired history professor who had been taking warfarin, vitamins, and minerals for a number of years, found that he was getting worn out easily and that he was often sweaty, exhausted, and lethargic. His doctor found that he was anemic and, with further tests, that his heart and spleen were both greatly enlarged. He gave Max several transfusions and took him off his vitamins and blood thinner. "While I was in the hospital, they didn't give me any blood thinner," he said. "They found no threat of harm in any of my vitamins or minerals, but they've asked me not to take the blood thinner because they thought it was the culprit. My doctor said, 'Maybe you needed a blood thinner when Dr. X prescribed it, but I doubt it. Certainly, you don't need it now. It's a *very dangerous* drug.'

"Knowing how cautious doctors have to be about accusing other doctors, I felt that he must have great suspicions about the blood-thinning ordeal I have lived through for six years. There was strong feeling in my doctor's voice when he expressed his view. He seemed angry and upset about what the other doctor had done, but of course, he didn't say it."

Ways to Offset Side Effects

Some other side effects that could cause harm or discomfort can be compensated for by your diet.

If you're taking a drug that makes you drowsy, for instance, you can take it at a time of day when you won't be driving. If a drug tends to be constipating, you can add bran, prunes, and roughage to your diet. Some drugs that upset your stomach should be taken with a glass of milk—but make sure it's okay with your doctor, since some medicines, and some antibiotics in particular, should not be taken with milk.

Coping with the side effects you experience is easier if you understand the peak levels of these drugs. For some drugs, when the drug is working the most actively in your system, you shouldn't be doing the most activity. It's particularly important to know about peak levels when you're taking insulin, for instance. When the level of insulin in your system peaks, your blood sugar will go down the most, and symptoms, such as your hands shaking, will appear. It's important, if you're a diabetic, to prepare for that drop in blood sugar by taking a snack along with you to eat if and when symptoms appear.

ADVERSE DRUG REACTIONS

Adverse drug reactions are one of the greatest health hazards for older people taking prescription or nonprescription drugs. These serious reactions to medications—which often happen after a slow accumulation of a drug becomes toxic—are often life-threatening. The World Health Organization defines these adverse drug reactions as "noxious and unintended."

Unfortunately, as we've pointed out previously, older people are much more likely to have adverse reactions than younger people because their bodies metabolize drugs more slowly and thus take longer to process medications from their systems. Older people also have an increased sensitivity to drugs. One study shows that seventy- to eighty-year-olds experience twice as many adverse reactions as forty- to fifty-year-olds. Even people fifty to fifty-nine are more likely than people ten years younger to become overmedicated.

A nightmare for many older people occurs all too often when an adverse drug reaction is incorrectly diagnosed as a new illness, for which the doctor prescribes yet another drug. This, of course, compounds the problem at a time when the doctor should be stopping or reducing the drug that actually is causing the "new illness." More often than not, that first drug is altogether unnecessary, should be given in smaller doses, or should be substituted for a safer drug.

Certainly, if you are on medication—even if you've been on it for many years—and you begin to feel dizzy and lose your balance, or become forgetful, delirious, confused, depressed, or downright crazy, suspect your medication first. This is also true if you lose your appetite, feel nauseated or constipated, have abdominal pain, or even have difficulty controlling your urine.

You may be on a medication that you've taken for years, but if your body is not functioning in the same way it used to, and if the drug is not excreted as readily, you probably have too much of the drug remaining in your system.

The drugs themselves have a period of time that it takes for one-half of the original maximum level of the drug in the blood to leave your system—a phenomenon called half-life. Some drugs remain in your body much longer than other drugs. Some reports on Valium, for instance, says that half of the full-dose level stays in your bloodstream for thirty to sixty hours. That means if you take Valium on Monday, you well may have some of that same drug in your system on Wednesday, and perhaps even Thursday. If you take a Valium every night, you keep adding that night's dose to whatever is still in your body from before.

Keep in mind that by staying informed and alert, you can avoid adverse drug reactions. At the least, if you have an adverse drug reaction, you can recognize it for what it is and get the help you need for it.

A Toxic Level

When George Spears began to act crazy, no one ever suspected a toxicity from Lanoxin, the digitalis preparation he'd been taking for his heart for nine years. George, an alert and easygoing eighty-three-year-old who had always had a terrific sense of humor, suddenly started acting bizarre, shouting belligerently and behaving in such erratic ways with his bowling team that he had to stop his twice-weekly bowling. At home he began fighting with his wife, throwing clothes out of his drawers, and storming around the house.

Early during the period of his confusion, George couldn't remember for sure whether he'd taken his Lanoxin. He was supposed to take it every morning and every evening, but he didn't know whether he had or not, so he'd take another.

"My personality changed," says George. "I didn't exactly get mean, but I got close to it." George's condition got so severe that his wife was unable to care for him. She and George's daughter, a nurse, took him to the University of Washington, where they made a videotape of him. George couldn't remember the names of his children or the name of the president of the United States. "They had me putting round pegs in square holes," he says.

George's daughter then took over the management of his medications. She cut down on the Lanoxin, and George began to improve. It still took him nearly three months to get back to normal. "When I got better and saw the videos, I couldn't believe it was me," George says. "I was a different person." Now George's daughter puts all his medication in envelopes that are dated for two-week periods. George, who's eighty-five, is back to bowling with his team and enjoying his wife's company.

The maintenance of the proper level of the drug so that it's effective, not toxic, is a delicate and critical concern. No matter how long you've been taking any particular medication, suspect it of funny business if you experience unexplained symptoms. You and your doctor can work together to find the answer to the problem.

PROBLEM DRUGS

Some of the most common side effects and adverse reactions come from the drugs that are most commonly used by older people. These include antihypertensive medicines, cardiovascular drugs such as digoxin and anticoagulants, antiarthritics, gastrointestinal drugs, and psychotropics such as tranquilizers, sleeping pills, and antidepressants.

In a large multicenter study conducted from 1973 to 1980, two groups of drugs were found to have caused nearly two-thirds of all adverse drug reactions. According to Dr. Peter Lamy, who conducted the study, these were:

* Drugs acting on the cardiovascular system—antihypertensives, digoxin, and the diuretics.
* Drugs acting on the central nervous system—psychotropics, anticholinergics, anti-parkinsonian drugs, and the hypnotics.

As Dr. Lamy points out in "Patterns of Prescribing and Drug Use" in *The Aging Process*, the fact of cardiovascular drugs and central nervous system drugs causing the majority of adverse drug reactions "is consistent with the hypothesis of altered drug action in the elderly, which identifies these two systems as exhibiting the greatest age-related changes. An examination of the top nine drugs used for the very old shows that four of the nine drugs belong to the class of drugs most frequently causing side effects." The side effects of all these drugs are significant. The numbers of older people on these drugs are significant. Statistics show, for instance, that 80 percent of all cardiovascular and antiarthritic drugs are prescribed for elderly patients.

High Blood Pressure Drugs
Many different medicines are used to treat hypertension. They work by making it easier for the blood to flow through the blood vessels and by reducing the volume of fluids in the body so that there is less pressure on the walls of the blood vessels. No *cure* has been found for hypertension, so the goal of treatment is to *control* it. Controlling it, however, requires a commitment. If you stop your medication when your blood pressure improves, it will go up again, and you will run the increased risk of heart failure, stroke, heart attack, or kidney failure. Several different kinds of antihypertensives that help lower the blood pressure are listed and described by the United States Pharmacopoeial

Convention in their book, *About Your High Blood Pressure Medicines*. They are:

- Beta-adrenergic blocking agents that help reduce the workload of the heart by affecting the response to some nerve impulses to the heart and blood vessels. Examples are acebutolol, atenolol, labetalol, metoprolol, nadolol, pindolol, propranolol, and timolol. (These are often not recommended for older people who have decreased cardiac output.)
- Calcium channel blocking agents that relax the blood vessels and reduce the workload of the heart by their effect on the movement of calcium into the cells of the heart and the blood vessels. Examples are diltiazem, nifedipine, and verapamil.
- Medicines such as hydralazine and minoxildil that act directly on blood vessels by relaxing them so that blood passes through them more easily.
- Medicines that act on the nervous system and relax blood vessels by controlling nerve impulses along certain nerve pathways. Examples are clonidine, guanabenz, guanadrel, guanethidine, methyldopa, pargyline, prazosin, and rauwolfia alkaloids.
- Angiotensin-converting enzyme (ACE) inhibitors such as captopril and enalapril that block an enzyme in the blood that causes blood vessels to tighten, and as a result, relax blood vessels.
- Diuretics or "water pills" that help reduce the amount of salt or water in the body by increasing the flow of urine. Examples of these pills are thiazide diuretics, loop diuretics, and potassium-sparing diuretics.

In addition to their benefits, most of these medicines have side effects, some of which are only bothersome and some of which are serious. Almost any one of the medicines listed may cause some degree of dizziness or light-headedness upon standing—a phenomenon called postural hypotension. The goal of treatment in high blood pressure, however, is to treat *without* side effects. Even when drugs are effective at lowering blood pressure, it's very important that dosages be adjusted to the individual's needs so that no side effects are experienced.

Digoxin and digitoxin, which are forms of digitalis, have a great number of side effects. The difference between an effective dose and a toxic dose of digitalis is very narrow. If you're having a toxic reaction to digitalis, you may lose your appetite, have diarrhea, or start throwing up. You may feel drowsy or have changes in your vision such as seeing spots or a halo around objects. Any potassium loss in your system makes your heart extremely sensitive to the toxic effects of digitalis. Irregular heartbeats and palpitations, confusion, or disorientation are red flags that you could be in serious trouble with a digitalis preparation, such as Lanoxin (digoxin). If you experience any adverse reaction, discontinue the medicine and call your doctor immediately.

Digoxin, which some reports say is used by 20 to 50 percent of the elderly in nursing homes, often leads to these adverse reactions. Digoxin is particularly hazardous because the margin between a safe dose and a toxic one is very narrow. Some studies have shown that certain patients who are receiving digoxin could safely be taken off it with no deleterious effects. Patients should never self-prescribe or take themselves off this drug, however. Any change should be thoroughly discussed with your doctor and made under his supervision.

Diuretics and vasodilators can have serious side effects that include electrolyte imbalance, depression, light-headedness, dizziness, or fainting. If you're experiencing problems from a diuretic, you may notice that you're thirsty, drowsy, weak, and lethargic. This may be due to shifts in the volume of the potassium

levels in your body. Other reactions due to shifts in
volume and low potassium include feeling restless and
fatigued, having cramps or weakness in your muscles,
and urinating less frequently.

The Public Citizen Health Research Group has found
that high blood pressure drugs containing reserpine (such
as Ser-ap-es, Diupres, and Hydropres) are dangerously
misprescribed for older adults. Their studies show that
reserpine can create serious drug-induced depressions.

Your doctor may give you one or two medications to
bring your blood pressure under control. It may be that
he won't try to make your blood pressure perfectly
"normal," but will let it remain slightly higher to avoid
side effects. If the dosage to bring your blood pressure
to normal keeps you dizzy or impotent, you'll probably
agree with him that the negative side effects outweigh
the benefits. It may be that you will have to stay in close
touch with him while he tries different medicines at
different dosages until he finds the combination that
works best for you.

Central Nervous System Drugs

Medications used to control pain or reduce inflammation affect the central nervous system. When they're
prescribed or taken incorrectly, these drugs often cause
adverse reactions in older people.

A large number of older people use antiarthritic medicines to control distress caused by arthritis or other
pains from joints in the fingers, legs, shoulders, hips,
or arms that have become swollen or inflamed. The pain
relievers and newer class of anti-inflammatory drugs
referred to as NSAIDS (Nonsteroidal Anti-inflammatory
Agents) used to control these problems include aspirin,
ibuprofen (Advil, Motrin, Nuprin, and Rufen), indomethacin (Indocin), sulindac (Clinoril), naproxen (Naprosyn), phenylbutazone (Butazolidin), piroxicam
(Feldene), and meclofenamate (Meclonen).

Any older person who uses daily doses of an anti-inflammatory drug should take it only under a doctor's supervision. This includes over-the-counter ibuprofen, which is said to be more gentle on the stomach than aspirin but can also cause problems if used for more than occasional relief. Too much of any anti-inflammatory drug can cause a skin rash, swollen face, itching, chills and fever, mild or severe stomach upset, blurry vision, light-headedness, diarrhea, nausea, and vomiting.

While aspirin and NSAIDS are effective in controlling pain, they're also irritating to the lining of the stomach and can adversely alter your kidney function or cause the development of stomach ulcers. According to the FDA, about two to four of every one hundred people taking these drugs will develop stomach ulcerations. Ulcers from aspirin and NSAIDS are particularly dangerous because these medications mask pain signals, and the ulcers tend to go undetected until they are bleeding and extremely serious.

Sucralfale (Carafate) is often prescribed in conjunction with NSAIDS to preserve the stomach. Another effective stomach-protecting drug, misoprostol (Cytotec), was approved in January 1989 by the FDA to prevent stomach damage from aspirin and NSAIDS. Cytotec is widely used in Europe and is only beginning to be used by doctors in the United States. It can cause diarrhea in the first few weeks of use, so a low dosage should be taken initially. Over-the-counter antacids that contain magnesium (such as Maalox or Mylanta) should **not** be taken along with the Cytotec. It is best to avoid antacid use and to take the drug with a meal, a snack, milk, or other liquids.

Adverse reactions to drugs that affect the central nervous system include oversedation (you are sleepy, groggy, and your speech may be slurred), impaired mental functioning (you get confused and forgetful), impaired gait (you don't walk normally), and hypoten-

sion (feeling dizzy or light-headed when you stand). All
of these reactions can lead to falls and hip fractures.

Pain relievers such as codeine sulfate, pentazocine
(Talwin), and demerol are controlled substances and are
especially dangerous if you are over sixty-five. If you
use these, you should be very careful; be sure to keep
your doctor informed about your reactions and the way
you are feeling. All these drugs can be habit-forming,
but if you take them for pain relief and they are effective, don't worry too much about dependency. When
the condition that's causing the pain goes away, some
pain experts say, so will your desire for the drug.

PEOPLE MOST AT RISK FOR ADRS

People who are most at risk when it comes to adverse
drug reactions, says Dr. Ron Adelman at Mount Sinai
Hospital, are people who have had previous drug reactions and people with a history of allergies. Other
people who fit the "at risk" profile for adverse drug
reactions include women of small stature, men or
women with liver or kidney disease, people with a history of mental problems, people with a history of visual
impairments, and people who have multiple diseases or
who are taking multiple drugs.

How can you tell if you're having an adverse reaction to a medicine? First of all, if you see yellow
halos around objects, or if you become dizzy, faint,
nauseated, or uninterested in food, suspect your
medication. Other clues that lead to the medicine
cabinet include stomach cramps, severe agitation, depression, or ringing in your ears. (Ringing in your
ears is often a sign that you're overdosing on aspirin.)
You may notice that you're losing your balance and
tripping over things, or that you've become confused,
depressed, forgetful, or irritable. You may be constipated, have diarrhea, or become incontinent, or it

may be that your face, arms, or legs start moving involuntarily.

No matter your symptoms, call your doctor and report your reactions. Tell him, "Since I've been taking *X*, I'm feeling dizzy" (describe whatever you're experiencing). Write down the ways you've been feeling before you call him so that you remember to include all the symptoms. Also tell him how you've been taking the prescription. Are you taking it exactly as prescribed? Any more? Any less? Truth is your ally. The details will help him determine just what is going on.

Some adverse drug reactions are not at all predictable because there isn't certainty as to how a person will react to a drug, even if she follows the drug regimen prescribed. Many adverse drug reactions *are* predictable, however. If the patient is informed about how to use the medicine and follows the physician's recommendations, more often than not an adverse drug reaction can be reversed with a dose adjustment. As we've said before, sometimes an ADR is the result of cumulative effects, and, even more often, the result of drug interactions or drug and food, or drug and alcohol interactions, many of which have slowly built up to toxic levels in the system. (This will be more thoroughly discussed in chapter 7.)

ALLERGIC REACTIONS

Allergic reactions usually happen to people who are hypersensitive to particular drugs almost immediately after taking them. These reactions usually occur within an hour—or sometimes within seconds or minutes of taking the drug. These two types of allergic reactions are called "delayed" or "immediate" reactions.

Allergic reactions are not subtle responses that can

be dealt with by the adjustment of dosage levels. They are extreme. They can come from ingesting drugs meant for external use or from taking even a minute amount of almost any kind of drug your body simply cannot tolerate. An allergic reaction can come from taking almost any medication, but according to *The Nurse's Guide to Drugs*, they're most likely when the drug is penicillin or some other antibiotic, immune serum, vaccine, toxoid, antitoxin, antivenin, sulfonamide, or when it is a drug used in a diagnostic skin test.

Symptoms of allergic reactions may include any one or several of the following:

- Coughing, wheezing, or the sensation of something closing up in your chest, and/or spasms of your bronchial tubes
- A feeling of swelling in the throat and/or difficulty breathing
- Uneasiness
- Agitation or loss of consciousness
- Rapid pulse, low blood pressure, fainting, arrhythmias (irregular pulse), shock, or cardiac arrest (the heart stops)
- Eye, ear, nose, and throat reactions—conjunctivitis, itchy or watery eyes, nasal congestion, and itching
- Gastrointestinal reactions—nausea, pain, vomiting, or diarrhea
- Skin reactions—flushing, a rash, itching, swelling, hives

Even when you are aware that certain complications and allergic reactions are uncommon, you should remember: 1) they happen, and 2) they can be dangerous. One of the biggest dangers of delayed allergic reactions happens when people don't suspect the medication they're on and seek treatment for a new disease. This happened in a minor way to Monica White's mother, who had been prescribed an antibiotic for a minor case of bronchitis. The antibiotic helped her feel better, but she got a rash. She called her daughter and asked her if she'd mind going with her to the dermatologist. She said she couldn't figure out why she had such a disturbing rash. Besides, she wanted it cleared up before a special dinner party she was attending on the weekend. Monica left work early to pick up her mother. In the car, right outside the dermatologist's office, she looked at her mother's skin eruptions. "Mother, I know what that is!" she exclaimed. "I've seen that before! Are you on antibiotics?" Her mother said yes, but the thought had never occurred to her that the rash might be related to her medicine. Instead of spending the time and the money going to a different doctor—probably to have been told it was a drug rash, or mistakenly to have received a second medication that could adversely interact with, or cancel, the effectiveness of her antibiotic—she called her first doctor and told him about the rash. He told her to stop taking the antibiotic. He changed her prescription, and the rash disappeared.

What to Do

If you have an allergic reaction to a medication, stop taking the drug immediately. If you have an immediate and severe reaction, call an ambulance, if necessary, or go straight to the nearest emergency room. Don't drive yourself. If you're alone, call a friend or neighbor over to help you or to stay with you until help arrives or your symptoms subside. If you go to the emergency room, take the medication with you. Make sure to loosen your collar and keep your airway clear. Lie down and elevate your legs.

If you've had allergic reactions to drugs before, you're a good candidate for having them again. Make sure to tell every doctor and dentist you see that you are allergic by nature and that you've had allergic

reactions to specific drugs before. Tell them the name
of those drugs and your specific reactions. There's no
point in going through repeat performances. If a doctor
is giving you a medication that you've never had before
and if you tend to be allergic, discuss the allergic reactions you've had previously and ask for the safest alternative. In certain instances, a skin test might be
helpful. That way, if you're going to be hypersensitive
to it, you'll have a slight swelling instead of a whole-
body reaction.

If you are allergic to penicillin or some other
drug that is life-threatening, get a Medic-Alert bracelet that contains the relevant information. Wear it in
case you are ever in a situation where you're not
able to tell attending physicians about your sensitivities. This could mean the difference between life and
death.

COMPLIANCE: A CRITICAL FACTOR

If the drug or the dosage you are on is making you sick,
let your doctor know immediately. Don't wait until you
get worse. Talk to your doctor about it and follow up
on the medicine.

As we've said before, physicians sometimes tend not
to tell patients about side effects because they don't want
them to be anxious or suggestible and develop symptoms that they otherwise might not have as a result of
being told the possibilities. This is the same argument
that's used against giving drug information sheets to
patients about their prescriptions; but there's no evidence to back up this view.

You don't have to have an allergic reaction before
you put in a call to your doctor or pharmacist with
questions about any reaction that concerns you.
Even if you are not sure about what's making you
feel sick, but you're on medication, check it out

with a professional. You may think you're experiencing a drug effect that is harmless, but you don't want to wait for an adverse reaction to prove yourself wrong.

CHAPTER 7

Polypharmacy—Your Body as "Drug Central"

"Laura's mother was getting really bad off, and it got hard to take care of her. She kept us up night and day. She couldn't keep track of time, and her mind seemed to be going. A lot of it was her medicines, but we didn't know that then. I was up every night giving her pills and syrups.

"At the time she was on daily doses of Aldactone, Oxpam, Bentyl, Mellaril, Pavabid, Mitrolan, Viscerol, and Lomotil. She also took Tylenol, Valium, Primatene mist, a cough syrup, Doxidan, Synalar, and Meprobamate and Marax as needed.

"The Viscerol went way up in price. That was the stomach medicine they gave her. I'd written a letter asking the doctor if he could help in some way. The costs of these medicines were so high, and we had to have the doctor's order to let us substitute generic drugs. At the least I thought maybe he could stop charging us for the prescriptions he wrote. He was charging her four dollars for each prescription. One month he wrote two new prescriptions and charged her eight dollars. That's one-third of her monthly income. Laura called and asked to talk to him, but he never returned the calls.

"It makes you feel real helpless. Like something's got to be done. Our old folks need help, and some-

times it feels like there's really nobody out there to
help 'em."
    —"ANDY JOHNSON," sixty-four, TALKING ABOUT HIS
        EIGHTY-SEVEN-YEAR-OLD MOTHER-IN-LAW

DRUGS AND MORE DRUGS

The more drugs you take, the more potential hazards
you will face in your daily life. According to the Consumer Federation of America, adverse reactions from
the multiple use of drugs cause more accidental deaths
among people over sixty-five than slipping in bathtubs
or showers, falling on stairs or uneven floors, or being
in car accidents.

A closer look might reveal that many of these other
fatal accidents were also the result of mixing medications that caused people to be groggy, to lack coordination, or to be so dizzy that they slipped and fell.

As we've said before, no matter what age you are,
the more drugs you take, the more chances you have of
getting severely sick from the powerful reciprocal actions that these drugs cause within the body. Studies
show that the frequency of adverse reactions in any person of any age increases in direct proportion to the
number of drugs taken. "My doctor's real good," says
Betty Stoner, a sixty-three-year-old who lives in Lan-
caster, Pennsylvania, with her husband, Marvin. "I get
a lot of different reactions to my medications, and he
always seems to know what's doing it. He has me on
sixteen different medications, and I guess I need them
all because when I had my heart attack, it did some
damage to my heart.

"Three or four days a week, it seems, when I get up
in the morning, I'm dizzy. He says that's because of the
medicine. It keeps my blood pressure down. Then about
eleven o'clock every morning, I get real hungry because my blood sugar drops. He tells me to eat more

breakfast, but even when I do, I'm still hungry at the same time. Now I've gotten arthritis from one of the medicines I'm taking, so he's had me cut down on it. All the time, something different crops up, and it's always because of the medication.''

Betty Stoner's doctor may be a likable person, but clearly he isn't aware that the sheer volume and mixture of the drugs he's prescribing are making life dreadfully uncomfortable, and potentially dangerous, for his patient.

Unfortunately, one of the most common reactions to multiple medications is confusion, which exacerbates existing problems. One stockbroker in New York, for instance, told me about a spur-of-the-moment visit he had made to Atlanta after an alarming telephone conversation with his father. His father, a former state court judge who had always been a fastidious model of logic and clarity, had been rambling and incoherent on the phone. Arriving in Atlanta, my friend found out that his father had had a minor heart attack and had left the hospital with five different medications. By the time his son got to him, the judge, who lived alone, could only identify one of the medicines and its purpose. He was trying to do what was good for himself, but his confusion from the medications was so great that he had no idea what pills he was taking, how often, or how many he had taken. Because of his son's intervention, the judge was in a weak but stable and coherent condition within twenty-four hours. The doctor, who had been entirely unaware of the judge's plight, took him off three of the medications and lowered the dosages of the two he considered essential. He asked the judge to call his office daily for the first week so he could assess the drugs' effects.

AN UNHOLY BONDING

It's critical to remember that everything in our bodies is chemical and has interactions with other chemicals we add to them.

Multiple drugs often cause multiple problems because an increased number of side effects come with each of them. These side effects can cause a variation in the absorption, the metabolism, and the distribution of each drug, and they can change one another's effects. It also makes sense that when we take two or more medicines, there's an increased chance that the bonding will go awry and that the drugs will adversely affect either the same or different physiological systems. If the drugs are at odds with each other, or if they combine to create an excessive effect, there's also an increased chance that they'll interfere with the normal functioning of those systems.

One way of conceptualizing the "bonding" of drugs is to think of a married couple who are monogamous. Just as a committed partner in a monogamous marriage is already "taken" and is unavailable for a new match, so are the electrons of one drug when they bond with another substance. There isn't room for another bonding or a real change of that basic unit. If, for instance, tetracycline bonds with milk, the drug changes form; it is no longer free to bind itself to anything else. In this case, it can no longer do what it was intended to do for the body to fight disease. In a larger context, when the drug binds itself to certain other substances and changes form, it has the capacity to affect many of the systems in our bodies. It may disperse throughout the system or get drawn to the wrong receptor sites.

Sometimes taking multiple drugs decreases the effectiveness of one or more of the medications. This reaction is difficult to detect since it can be mistaken for a worsening of the disease or for the suspicion that a drug has failed to be effective.

Mixing Is Not Always Harmful

If you are taking three or four medicines—or if your parent is—don't become instantly alarmed from reading that multiple drug interactions have the potential to cause death. You may well be one of a vast number of your peers who *needs* several prescriptions to address your different physiological conditions. Most likely, the prescription medications you're taking are reasonable and legitimate and are based on judicious medical decision making. Sometimes three or four or even six drugs can be used effectively to manage chronic diseases and make you feel better. If you take them as you're supposed to, you're not likely to run into any high drama from adverse reactions.

It's not unusual for anyone over sixty to be taking multiple medications and managing them without any difficulty. It's not only very sick people who take a lot of medicine.

When I checked with my own mother, for instance, I was amazed to learn that her drug regimen definitely qualifies as "polypharmacy." I would never have thought of her as taking multiple medications because she's a vital, independent, and contented seventy-four-year-old. Although she had a hip replacement due to arthritis three years ago, and has ongoing high blood pressure, these things don't slow her down. She goes to the library, art museums, plays, and movies. She takes an active role in her church and her community. Nevertheless, she takes multiple medications on a tightly controlled schedule to address her multiple conditions. Every day she takes:

- Forty milligrams of Corgard, a beta-blocker to lower her blood pressure
- One two-grain thyroid pill
- Two tablets of Dyazide, an antihypertensive diuretic
- Estrogen (she takes tablets every three days)
- Two ten-grain coated aspirin for her arthritis

- Three hundred milligrams of Noludar, a sleeping pill
- Twenty meg K-Lor (potassium)
- Calcium
- Vitamin E
- Vitamin C
- Theragran-M
- Vitamin B_6 and
- Vitamin B_{12}

Although she takes more vitamins and prescription drugs than most geriatric physicians would recommend, her doctor has worked carefully with her to establish dosages that work best to treat her conditions without side effects. I've questioned her use of sleeping pills, but she takes them for anxiety-free sleeping and believes they don't cause her any problems. She's very careful about the way she takes all of her medications, and she points out that she never takes more or less than she's supposed to, and she takes them on schedule. She keeps her doctor informed of everything she's taking, questions him about anything new, *and* uses the *Physicians' Desk Reference, The Essential Guide to Prescription Drugs,* and *The Merck Manual* for reference. She's never had any adverse drug reactions, and I hope she never will.

Some people, however, haven't been so careful or so fortunate when it comes to multiple medications and their adverse interactions. It's estimated that 1.5 million people in the United States are hospitalized each year as a result of adverse drug reactions. From 10 to 25 percent of hospital admissions for the elderly are related to the effects of drugs. One study at University Hospital in Boston showed that out of 815 random admissions to the hospital, 33 percent had complications from treatment by their physicians. Although the data aren't definitive, researchers believe that at least 2 to 3 percent of the older population dies from adverse drug reactions or interactions. This represents a large number of people and thousands of deaths that could have—and should have—been avoided.

AVOIDABLE DEATHS

When deaths are clearly attributable to adverse drug reactions, studies show that death was due more to a multiplicity of drug use than to the age and sex of the victims.

The effects of drugs, however, may also be altered considerably because of health, age, diet, and disease. For instance, anticoagulants are said to be a major cause of death among the elderly due to adverse reactions. Yet, it may be that many of these deaths were related to the role of advanced heart disease and fatal illnesses that might have occurred even earlier without the drugs that eventually created those toxic reactions. Even the experts disagree on just how these deaths might have been avoided. Dr. James Long points out in *The Essential Guide to Prescription Drugs* that the true dimensions of the problem have not been established by research. According to Dr. Long, "Considered in the context of national drug consumption, serious adverse reactions are relatively uncommon. The majority of life-threatening drug reactions occur in people who are already severely ill with advanced or known fatal disease. Most serious adverse reactions are caused by a small number of drugs which are quite hazardous by nature, and the number of deaths properly attributed to drugs is quite small in relation to the number of lives saved by these same drugs."

In making the decision to use a toxic drug, doctors have to decide whether the possible benefits of the drugs outweigh the risks by a considerable margin. "If someone has cancer, you give him chemotherapy, which is poison," says Dr. Michael Freedman at New York University Medical Center. "But when you weigh the risk against one hundred percent death, it's worth taking it. If the risk is that 50 percent of the time it's going to save the patient, it's worth taking it. Even if it's a 10 or 20 percent chance to save the patient, it's worth it when there's no alternative. Some of the medicines that are given that are the *worst* medicines are given because the circumstances are so terrible.

"Where doctors make mistakes is when they give medicines for a condition that isn't particularly life-threatening. Then, the risks begin to outweigh the benefits. For instance, if you give medicines to protect a ninety-year-old from the long-term risks of hypertension and that medicine causes the patient to be dizzy and risk falling, then the benefits aren't worth it. It may be better to have the blood pressure slightly higher than normal and not take risks of fatal falls."

According to the director of the Center for the Study of Pharmacy and Therapeutics for the Elderly at the University of Maryland, Dr. Peter Lamy, most of the deaths that result when risks outweigh the benefits should never occur.

"From a statistical point of view, it's true that serious or fatal adverse reactions are relatively uncommon," says Dr. Lamy. But he insists that even 2 or 3 percent of the older population dying from adverse drug reactions is far too high, particularly, he says, since most of those deaths were avoidable.

"We shouldn't pat ourselves on the back and say it's only 2 or 3 percent who die from adverse drug reactions! That's too many!"

The Hidden Statistics

Assessing the incidence and consequences of adverse drug reactions due to drug interactions is very difficult. The real "proof" of any adverse reaction depends on the disappearance of the adverse reaction when the drug is withdrawn and its reappearance when begun again.

Open-and-shut cases of the casual relationship between drugs and death are difficult to prove.

According to the *The Merck Manual* the most commonly reported causes of drug-related deaths are:

- Gastrointestinal hemorrhage from peptic ulceration—corticosteroids, aspirin, and other anti-inflammatory drugs and anticoagulants
- Other hemorrhages—anticoagulants, and drugs used to treat cancer
- Aplastic anemia—chloramphenicol, phenylbutazone, gold salts
- Hepatic damage—chlorpromazine, isoniazid
- Renal failure—analgesics
- Infection—corticosteroids, cytostatic drugs
- Anaphylaxis—penicillin, antiserums

Many of these drugs are used in life-threatening situations by doctors who determine the risks are necessary and advisable in their efforts to save a life.

While there may not be a definitive analysis or even an awareness of all the mortalities related to adverse reactions or interactions, you can deduce from looking at case records that drugs have been the major contributing factor in many serious illnesses and deaths. Even when it's quite easy to deduce the toxicities of drugs, however, a death will rarely be ascribed to drugs. Dr. Lamy points out, for instance, that a large number of people over sixty-five die of incidents related to peptic ulcers, compared with a small percentage under sixty-five. We know, he says, that the peptic ulcers are related to adverse reactions to substances such as aspirin, but it's not documented. In a similar way, if a doctor gives a patient an antidepressant, morphine, and another drug that together induce a brain problem, many people will not be looking at the death as the result of a drug interaction, nor will most doctors draw attention to a drug-induced death even if they are aware of it.

"Drug-induced renal failure will probably never be observed either," says Dr. Lamy. "It starts quietly and then it's suddenly over!" Fatal combinations of drugs often aren't officially labeled as such—because the more immediate "cause of death" is cardiac arrest or the shutting down of some other system. Because we don't look for adverse drug reactions, we often don't think about what has actually triggered the action that caused the fatality.

"Durant Wheeler" 's death was attributed to his heart. But anyone thinking about drug toxicity would realize that the source of his death was the adverse interactions of medications used to treat him. Mr. Wheeler, a real-estate owner in Los Angeles, had rarely had a cold, let alone any major illness. An active seventy-six-year-old who often made repairs and walked around the apartment buildings he owned with a wrench and screwdriver sticking out of his back pocket, he had severe chest pains one day and was admitted to the hospital. While he was there, his doctor gave him a diuretic. Another doctor, seeing the prescription for Lasix on Mr. Wheeler's chart, prescribed liquid potassium to balance the Lasix—which would not be inappropriate if careful measurements of renal function and potassium levels in the blood had been made. This, however, was not the case with Mr. Wheeler, who was not monitored. Moreover, he was sent home with additional liquid potassium by a third doctor. Within four days after going home from the hospital, a critically ill Mr. Wheeler was back in the hospital as a result of a critical imbalance of medications, which led within a few days to his death, diagnosed as cardiac arrest.

In another person, the same amount of potassium might not have been an overdose. But when it comes to medications, the margin of safety with dosages is sometimes a critical matter.

The Danger of More Than One Physician

Unfortunately, Durant Wheeler's case is not unusual. Because it's often necessary for people to be seen by more than one specialist in addition to their regular physician, problems arise because one doctor is unaware of what another has prescribed. "Tom Latimer," a retired builder, says he got into trouble when his hay fever started acting up. He called his internist and asked him for a prescription for an antihistamine. It never occurred to him to tell his doctor that he was still taking Valium, an antianxiety medication, prescribed by the psychiatrist he had started seeing when he was feeling very depressed shortly after retirement. He picked up the antihistamine at a drugstore and never thought to tell his pharmacist about it. (His pharmacist kept records on him and would have been able to warn him of the interactive effects of the antihistamine and Valium.) "I started feeling really low and basically suicidal," Tom says. "I don't think I would have figured it out if I hadn't run out of Valium and called my doctor to see if he could give me another prescription for it. He said that the antihistamine and the anxiolytic [antianxiety] were almost bound to make me chemically depressed in an excessive way. You just don't realize that those emotions are chemical because they *feel* so real."

"An older couple in Kansas are typical of many people who get into trouble with multiple diseases, multiple physicians, and multiple medications. Dale Sorenson, a retired farmer and his wife, "Ruby," have to drive forty miles to get lab work done. They drive two and a half hours to see their family doctor and their orthopedic doctor and, for more serious matters, such as Dale's heart, they drive to the state capital, which eats up their entire day. At one point, when Dale had hip surgery, his surgeon put him on two different medications. His heart doctor had him on three other kinds of medicine.

"We became really alarmed when we found out he

was taking nine medicines a day,'' said ''Janice Weston,'' Dale's daughter-in-law. ''From what we understood, doctors can't tell you the interactions of more than three medications at a time. You're just out there in the woods experimenting. And yet the specialists seemed reticent to manipulate medications prescribed by a doctor in a different area.

''We got real concerned because Dad got so lethargic. We were wondering how much it was because of the combination of these medications. We said, 'Take these medicines in and ask the doctor,' but we haven't gotten satisfactory answers from the doctor.

''Dad was given medicine to take regularly and medicine to take in case of a particular symptom. For instance, he was given nitroglycerin patches to apply regularly and nitroglycerin to take in case of chest pains. Since he's so far from the doctor who set this up, he's not under constant supervision, so every time he felt alarmed or concerned about his heart, he'd put on a nitroglycerin patch. It turned out that he was doing it all the time, and he was only supposed to be applying it once a day. At one point he was walking, and he felt really bad. He sat down, and Mother came by and saw that he looked really white. She took him down to the doctor, and his blood pressure was way down. He had almost no pulse.

''They found out that he was compounding the regular heart medicine he was taking with the nitroglycerin. When I looked into it, I found out about a therapy program for heart patients for follow-up and follow-through. Things apparently often get confused when people are predisposed not to take pills or when they depend too heavily on them and then double up on their prescriptions. Unless they're monitored, it's hard to get them to take the right amount of medication.''

168   THE SAFE MEDICINE BOOK

Overly Aggressive Treatment

According to Dr. Peter Lamy, there are strong indications that many older patients under long-term care receive drug treatment when there may be no indication
for its need. This stems from the fact that long-term,
chronic-care is rooted in the problem-solving methods
used for acute care. "In acute care, success is equated
with a short-stay institutionalization and complete recovery," he says. "Acute care often involves intense
use of drugs, frequent and probable overuse of diagnostic procedures, use of high-cost technology and
high-cost systems, and disregard for the influence of
family and such concerns as the patient's nutritional
status." What is needed in long-term care, Dr. Lamy
says, is management of long-term ailments with the
*least interference possible in the older person's func-
tioning on all levels.*

Sometimes it seems that in a futile, if not frantic,
attempt to "cure" instead of "manage" a condition
that's bound to be persistent and long-lasting, doctors
lose sight of the full life of their older patient. It's vital
to an older person, just as it is to a younger one, to
operate at maximum level. If a person is slowed down
or debilitated by a disease, then adjustments need to be
made to enhance his life, not diminish it further. Yet
some doctors give the patient multiple drugs that unnecessarily interfere with vision, mobility, mental
coherence, and emotional and physical stability.

In " Agnes Miller" 's case, her doctor of thirty years
adamantly and often rudely defended the fifteen prescriptions he had ordered for her despite the fact that
they were making her sick. He seemed to have little
regard for helping Mrs. Miller live the best life possible. He demonstrated this most profoundly by disclaim-
ing and disregarding the realities of Agnes's
deteriorating personality and ability to function—a phenomenon painfully obvious to Agnes's daughter and son-
in-law, "Laura and Andy Johnson."

Laura's mother, Agnes, was eighty-seven when she came to live with sixty-one-year-old Laura and her husband, Andy, sixty-four, in their home in a small Nebraska town. Agnes had been in a nursing home for a year following a broken hip, and Laura and Andy felt they could care for her better at home. Agnes had always been lively and active, but when she came home, she was sick, sluggish, and miserable.

"She had a list of medicines a foot long," Andy recalls. "She was on medications for nerves, medications to help her sleep, to adjust her system, to adjust her regularity with her bowels, for throat spasms, for indigestion, and for a hiatus hernia. We wanted to find out if the doctor could cut out some of them. He was irate. He wouldn't change anything.

"I'd say he was uncooperative. But Agnes liked that doctor. She'd had him for years and years, so that's the reason we kept him. I tried to keep track of the medicines by reading about them and looking at these TV shows where they would discuss them. We heard a report on one show that this one medicine she was taking was real harmful, and they were taking it off the market. We asked her doctor about it, but he said she had to have it and he wouldn't take her off it. Then, lo and behold, they took it off the market and he had to drop it off her list.

"Laura's mother was getting really bad off, and it got hard to take care of her. She kept us up night and day. She couldn't keep track of time, and her mind seemed to be going. A lot of that was because of her medicines, but we didn't know that then. I was up every night giving her the medicines. There were eight or nine different ones I had to give her during the night—not even counting the daytime ones.

"Finally we had to take her back to the nursing home. We moved and got work nearby there so that we could be close to her. We wanted to cut back on costs. There was only one pharmacy in town, and that druggist wouldn't give out generics. He was the same person who sold the medicines to the nursing home, so nobody got a break.

"We did get her off Mellaril with the help of a nurse from the nursing home. That happened when we brought her home for a weekend. We gave her Mellaril, and she went completely berserk. We told the nurse what happened, and she talked to the doctor and got her off that. Right away we all noticed improvement. We also noticed that when she took Pavabid, she would become irritable, disoriented, and negative. Her doctor wouldn't budge on cutting back Pavabid or any of her other medicines, and then one time, when she fell, he wouldn't even go out to look at her hip or have it X-rayed until we insisted. He just wouldn't do common-sense things for her, and it got so that he wouldn't even return our telephone calls.

"So, finally, we got her to agree to change doctors. This new doctor sees Agnes once a month, and he shows an interest in her. He said he'd try taking her off the Pavabid, and he did. She never had any problem from being off it, and in fact, she felt better. Now she's off the Oxpam, Mellaril, Pavabid, Mitrolan, and Gaviscon. He said that if she needs an antacid, she can take Maalox Plus. She's more like herself again."

CREATING NEW ILLNESSES

Many times doctors are unaware that they're creating illnesses in their own patients. They keep adding medicines to deal with all the new symptoms of diseases that are being produced—deepening the effect and making the patient sicker all the time. This phenomenon is often referred to as an "illness-medication spiral."

Testifying at hearings conducted by the Joint Subcommittee on Health and Long-Term Care of the Aging, Mrs. Rose Zimny of Everett, Massachusetts, said that in 1980, her mother, Gloria Zimny, saw a well-regarded internist who prescribed steroids to treat an asthmatic condition. When her condition worsened, the doctor kept her on the steroids and prescribed more medicine. By August 1981, she was taking ten to twelve prescribed drugs daily.

"My mother [who was only sixty-five at the time] was showing some signs of memory loss and became very nervous and agitated," said Rose Zimny. "About the second or third week of November, she had the worst attack of all. Nothing seemed to help her breathe. I brought her to the same doctor because I figured he knew her history and would be able to treat her better. This time the doctor put her in the hospital and started giving her high doses of everything to try to control her breathing, and nothing would work. . . . After three weeks of visiting her, I started to notice that she was talking when nobody was there and praying to God to please let somebody help her because the doctor she had placed all her trust in was trying to kill her. . . .

"She was also unable to walk and had severe heart palpitations. Her doctor was away every weekend, and it became increasingly difficult to reach him. On the twenty-fifth, I received a phone call from the doctor, and my mother was screaming in the background. I asked him what was wrong, and he said, 'I think you had better come over here, because she is going crazy.' . . . He tried to blame it on an upset in her life, but I told him that was ridiculous. I had seen her upset before, but she was now hysterical. . . . He sent in a psychiatrist, who agreed with what he had said.

"Eventually I insisted that he release her, and he did, sending her home with about twenty different prescriptions. He felt he was doing nothing wrong, but he was killing her slowly. While she was home, she knew exactly when it was time to take her pills and screamed in horror just looking at the bottles. I knew then it was the pills doing this to my mother."

After seeing her mother go through several more episodes of fainting, slipping in and out of comas, and being admitted for emergency treatment to a different Boston hospital, Rose Zimny was finally referred to Dr. Jonathan D. Lieff at Lemuel Shattuck Hospital in Jamaica Plains, Massachusetts.

"When I arrived with my mother, I explained to him what was happening, and he was very understanding," said Rose Zimny. "He arranged for me to stay with my mother because she was so afraid of being left alone. Dr. Lieff and a colleague of his named Dr. Zubaragu immediately took the pills away from her. Within four days, she was starting to walk and act exactly like herself. I will always feel that if it wasn't for these doctors, she might not be here today."

In discussing this case, Dr. Lieff said that Mrs. Zimny's case, unfortunately, is all too common. He said they had given Mrs. Zimny what they call "the plastic bag test"—asking her to put all the medications she was taking into a plastic bag. "She had been given groups of medicines from two different sources," he said, "and some of them were overlapping. But basically, there were medicines for asthma, steroids; then sleeping pills, anxiety pills, tranquilizers; antacids for indigestion, which was caused by some of the medicines; cardiac medications and potassium, because of side effects from other medication. So, the medicines created a vicious cycle. She started having tachycardia and from there ended up with cardiac medicines. One thing led to another, until she had the twenty-two medicines at that time."

The physician who prescribes twenty-two medications should know better. But it's also true that consumers should know better as well. There are, however, a lot of different ways that people of all ages, but particularly older people, get themselves on multiple prescriptions without considering the potential damage. Some of these ways include:

- Accumulating doctors and prescriptions and not telling the next doctor you see about the other doctors or the other prescriptions.
- Failing to tell your doctor what other nonprescription medications you're taking, such as aspirin, vitamins, and laxatives.
- Using medicines you've stored up, or one you used for ''something similar'' a while back. In this way, you're adding your own ''prescription'' to the process.
- Trading or borrowing medications from a friend.

By taking a doctor's prescription without telling her about the drug regime you are already on, you're sabotaging her efforts and putting yourself in a dangerous situation. If the doctor doesn't have a clue as to how many medicines you are taking, she may think she's seeing a new disease that needs treatment.

One Extreme
Recently, a good friend of mine was telling me about her twenty-year-old son, who was home from college with mononucleosis. ''Jason loves pills,'' she said. ''Honestly, he's an amateur pharmacist! He doesn't know the meaning of discomfort without taking a pill. For a while he had a series of infections, so he took antibiotics. First he came home with six little pills wrapped in brown paper with no label on them at all. Someone had just written on the outside of the paper to take three a day. Jason—he does know to ask questions—told me, 'This is a synthetic penicillin, which will act quickly on the bacterial infection!' I was so upset that he was taking prednisone, and that it wasn't labeled. . . . I called the doctor and he convinced me that it would be helpful.

''When he went in to see the doctor again last week, the doctor gave him Novahistine for his little cough and

eye drops for his puffy eyes. Look, I understand. There's
no doctor who sends you out of his office without a
prescription in your hand—and these are good doctors.
But still . . . Now he's taken Tylenol nonstop for two
weeks. Finally he got a stomachache from it. He called
the doctor, and the doctor gave him Donnatal. It stops
the peristalsis of the stomach, naturally, so he gets constipated. The doctor tells him to drink prune juice. He's
had so much prune juice now that the next thing you
know, he's going to be running out to get Maalox.

"This morning he had a headache and he asked me
for an aspirin, and I said, 'Why don't you just take the
whole medicine cabinet?' Every time I say he shouldn't
be taking something, he acts like I'm trying to kill
him.''

This woman was not talking about an aging parent
or an aging husband. Although twenty-year-old Jason's
way of turning to pills as the panacea of all discomforts
could apply to a person of any age, it's clear that we
sometimes form unhealthy dependencies on medicines
early—and don't break those habits before it's too late.

Medicine as Magic

Some people are so afraid of the effects of pills that
they refuse to take anything, even medicines that would
actually help them extend their lives or enhance their
feeling of well-being. But it seems as if a lot more of
us think of medicine—any medicine—as magic. Without understanding what we're doing, we become true
believers. It's just, "Take this; it's magic, it will make
you feel better!"

"It's okay to have that attitude that the medicine will
help," says Dr. Bernard Mehl of Mount Sinai. "If you
think of a pill as magic, that's not all bad. In fact, it
can be of use. Many studies have shown that placebo
medicine does have an effect. It may take away pain if
people believe in it. If you have the opposite attitude,

that it won't help a bit or that there's no magic here, that may not be helpful at all.''

Many of us, however, carelessly, and needlessly expose ourselves to risks when it comes to medications.

Every drug we take, no matter how minor it seems, has an effect on our bodies. It's easy to forget that fact and take them lightly. Too many people feel that there must be a pill to answer the problem each time they feel bad.

''Everybody forgets the delicacy of the human body,'' says a forty-six-year-old from Scarsdale, New York, who has been involved with a variety of medical problems in her family for many years. ''The doctors don't make you aware of what you're taking and how much of an effect it can have on you! And if you're like my sister-in-law, you think that the answer to every problem is in a bottle of pills! Her house looks like a pharmacy!''

It's because of that sort of thinking that we get into so much trouble with multiple use of drugs.

THE PHYSICIAN'S ROLE

No one understands all the possible combinations that can be harmful in any individual—and perhaps expecting the physician to know them all is unrealistic. There are always matters beyond a physician's control. For instance, sometimes a person takes a ''very safe drug'' and then dies from it. There's no possible way for the doctor to predict such an extreme response to what is considered a safe medication.

''I think it's literally impossible for physicians to keep up today with the information explosion,'' said Dr. Jonathan D. Lieff, director of Psychiatry and chief of Geriatrics at the Lemuel Shattuck Hospital in Jamaica Plains, Massachusetts, when he testified in 1983 before a Joint Subcommittee hearing on the health and long-term care of the aging. ''If you just look at aspirin alone

and try to memorize the number of other drug interactions with aspirin, there are twenty-five *known*
interactions with aspirin. . . . Yet, every single over-
the-counter medicine and every single prescription
medicine has interactions and has side effects interacting with many diseases. It is literally impossible for a
doctor to keep up.''

Aggressive monitoring of medications might help, but
few physicians have the time or energy for it. Often they
learn about adverse combinations only after it's too late
for the patient!

''As long as we're not thinking of adverse drug effects and interactions, we're not going to see them,''
says Dr. Lamy. ''Some of our findings have been ser-
endipitous. For instance, we used quinidine and digoxin
together for twenty-five years before we found out we
were giving it at toxic levels. Once it was possible to
measure the level in the blood, we learned that we
were giving doses that were too high. Now we know
that patients on this combination must have their blood
levels monitored frequently.''

Even with the massive amount of information provided, and even with what is still *not* known, however, Dr. Lamy says that *if doctors used what they knew,
almost all adverse drug interactions could be stopped.*
Dr. Lamy points to a study conducted at the Royal Liv-
erpool Hospital, where researchers reviewed cases of
adverse drug actions and interactions and found that 68
percent of the cases were avoidable and another 18 percent were probably avoidable ''had we used what we
know!''

''If I have a patient on an anticoagulant and I give
him cimetidine [Tagamet], I induce some drug interactions,'' says Dr. Lamy. ''I shouldn't use cimetidine,
I know that. But we're so used to using cimetidine that
it probably happens.

''If we read reliable research that tells us there may
be an association between depression and propranolol

use, we know that and shouldn't be using propranolol in those kinds of cases. If someone says there's a lot of depression caused by cimetidine if the dose is not adjusted, we know we must carefully titrate the dose. If we just used what we knew, we wouldn't have that many problems!''

Additionally, says Dr. Lamy, ''Long-term care ought to have different goals. The therapeutic goal should be one of care rather than cure. Disease management should take priority over cure. Realistic goals should include the effort *not* to decrease further a patient's already diminished quality of life and not to adversely affect a patient's physical, physiological, nutritional, functional, and mental status.''

Keep Your Caretakers Informed

If you're about to add another medication to your drug regimen, or you're currently taking two or more medicines, be alert to what you're doing. Learn about the benefits you should get from your drugs—and the precautions you should take. Make sure that your doctor knows what other medications—prescribed and not prescribed—you're using.

Mainly, remember that when your body is a central warehouse for chemicals, you must act as commander in chief and maintain control of what you put into it. Know what you're taking and ask your doctor how this drug will interact with your other medications. Remember, most difficulties of drug interactions can be avoided entirely if you and your doctor work together. You can't be too careful.

CHAPTER 8

Drugs in Disguise—Food, Alcohol, and Drug Combinations

"Round the neck of the bottle was a paper label, with the words 'Drink me' beautifully printed on it in large letters. It was all very well to say 'Drink me,' but the wise little Alice was not going to do *that* in a hurry. 'No, I'll look first,' she said, 'and see whether it's marked "poison" or not'; for she had read several nice little histories about children who had got burnt, and eaten up by wild beasts and other unpleasant things, all because they *would* not remember the simple rules their friends had taught them; such as, that a red-hot poker will burn you if you hold it too long . . . and she had never forgotten that if you drink much from a bottle marked 'poison,' it is almost certain to disagree with you, sooner or later.

"However, this bottle was *not* marked 'poison' so Alice ventured to taste it, and finding it very nice (it had, in fact, a sort of mixed flavor of cherry tart, custard, pineapple, roast turkey, toffee and hot buttered toast), she very soon finished it off."

—LEWIS CARROLL *Alice's Adventures in Wonderland*

When you eat cheese, does it ever occur to you that in combination with certain antibiotics it can be dangerous? Before you drink a cup of coffee, do you take stock of how it will interact with your heart medicine?

In recent years, we've all become more aware that certain foods affect our health. We realize, for instance, that there's an interrelationship between cholesterol and the heart and cholesterol levels and hypertension. We've learned that we should eat more fish and chicken and less red meat. News stories continue to inform us about recent suspicions or discoveries of food-disease relationships. For instance, it was recently discovered that raw mushrooms caused cancer in rats. We humans were advised to avoid eating mushrooms raw and told that it's preferable to eat them in soups, stews, or cooked as a side dish.

Despite more media coverage of these food and health issues, however, it's easy not to think of foods and beverages as drugs. Yet, according to pharmacists, a broad definition of drugs includes anything that affects the body—and this includes foods and beverages. It's easy, like Alice, to eat or drink something *not* marked "poison," and like her, sometimes only moments later say, "Curious!" as you hold onto your head and feel strange inside. Sometimes when you swallow something that you'd normally never be concerned about, you find yourself feeling peculiar and you don't know why. If you have such a reaction, it may be directly due to the interactive effects of certain foods you eat with certain medicines you're taking.

At the least, the effectiveness of your medicine can be offset by combining it with different foods or drinks or over-the-counter drugs you'd normally think of as harmless. At the worst, some of these drug interactions are life-threatening, so it's extremely important to find out from your doctor what should or should not be taken with your medicine.

For instance, under normal conditions, it can be great to sit down with a glass of wine and a plate of Brie or Cheddar cheese and crackers before dinner. But if you're a person who is being treated for depression with a drug such as tranylexpromine (Parnate), you should *never* eat these two particular cheeses or drink beer, vermouth, chianti, or sherry wines because the results could be anything but pleasurable and relaxing. That's because these cheeses and drinks contain a chemical that combines negatively with the antidepressant you're taking. The chemical in question, called tyramine, is also present in chicken liver, sour cream, salami, bologna, avocados, ripe bananas, raisins, and some other high-protein foods that have been aged or have undergone a breakdown process. Tyramine, which is converted into adrenaline by the body, has the capacity to raise your blood pressure. Under normal conditions, that elevation in your blood pressure is neutralized by certain enzymes called monoamine oxidases (MAO), which are found in your body tissues and function to metabolize noradrenaline.

Problems set in if you're taking drugs such as Eutonyl, Furoxone, Marplan, Nardil (phenelzine sulfate), or Parnate, which *block* the action of monoamine oxidase in your body. Such drugs (called MAO inhibitors) may be prescribed for severe depression that is chemically or biologically based. When the monamine oxidase is blocked, the actions of substances such as tyramine go unopposed, and relatively small amounts can cause dangerous elevations of blood pressure. In severe cases, the results can be fatal because the blood pressure increases to a critical point causing the vessels in the brain to break, resulting in cerebral hemorrhage.

Because these drugs are so dangerous, doctors usually prescribe them only when other, "safer" drugs have been ineffective, and they monitor them carefully. Still, if you're taking one of these MAO inhibitors, you should remember to avoid foods and beverages that contain tyramine.

There's a long list of what could be called unkind interactions between food and drugs. Over time, research will probably document, with precision, other problematic food and drug combinations. Some research is now pointing to the possibility that anticoagulants *may* have a direct interaction with certain green vegetables that contain phytic acid. Studies suggest that the phytic acid in spinach, kale, and broccoli can offset the effects of Coumadin.

If you are taking any drug on a regular basis, you should find out about its "drug-nutrient interactions." This means you should find out about the effect of the drug on your foods, and the effect of your foods and beverages on the way the drug is metabolized. Depending on what drug you're taking, your diet may need to include extra vitamins and minerals that are excreted because of the medicine. The importance of knowing the nutritional effects of medicines on your diet shouldn't be underestimated. In some states it's a requirement of hospital licensing that patients be notified of any potential drug-nutrient interactions when they leave the hospital.

When patients taking medications for arthritis leave a hospital in Maryland, for instance, they're told that their long-term use of anti-inflammatory steroids may cause a loss of calcium, and that they should add a certain amount of calcium to their diet to make up for that loss. If they're taking nonsteroidal anti-inflammatory agents, they are informed that medications such as ibuprofen have caused a variety of gastric problems and must *not* be taken on an empty stomach. Patients on antihypertensives are told, depending on the medication, that they may need to supplement their diet with extra potassium, magnesium, zinc, and perhaps calcium. And people taking tricyclic antidepressants are told that their drugs may affect glucose metabolism, which could cause them to eat more or make them so lethargic that they'll eat less. Along with the warnings and precautions, they're given advice on preventing complications and keeping themselves in good health.

Because drug-nutrient interactions are very complicated, it's important for the patient to find out what his

or her particular situation requires. The factors affecting
the way your food and medication interact include your
diet, your medication, what other medications you're
taking, (including over-the-counter drugs), your alcohol
consumption, your exercise patterns, and your own particular metabolism. If you are taking any medications
on a long-term basis, it would be a good idea for you
to find a registered dietitian who does nutritional counseling. Many times these counselors can be found
through your doctor or hospital, and they can help you
set up a diet that compensates for any losses due to the
medications and help you maintain healthy eating patterns that prevent further problems.

"INNOCUOUS" SUBSTANCES

Sometimes a well-meaning friend may offer you a drink
that a nutritionist recommended for her. "Here, drink
this! It will make you feel better," she might say. "It
always gives me a lot of pep." What she might not
know is that this drink may be high in potassium and
you may not need potassium. In fact, it may react very
badly with your potassium-sparing diuretic. Or it may
be that you're diabetic and the drink has too much sugar
in it. Potentially, her health drink could make you very
sick. Remember that what balances your system can
wreak havoc on another's.

Your nutritional requirements change as you get older.
You may be eating high protein and vegetables when
you need more carbohydrates in your diet. Don't prescribe your diet for your friends. If you want to be helpful, recommend that they go for their own analysis and
nutritional evaluation.

You might be naturally wary of a friend's "nutritional" drink, but what about the culprits in your everyday diet? Two common substances that many of us
consume as if they were harmless are sodium and caf-

feine. Masked within the daily rituals of our experiences, we hardly acknowledge them as drugs. The sodium can be found in the salt shakers on our tables, and the caffeine in the cups of coffee and tea over which we carry on our conversations.

Salt

When you pick up the salt shaker, do you think about the fact that you're adding sodium and chlorine to your body?

Since scientific research has linked excessive salt intake to hypertension and has established that consuming less sodium can help prevent and alleviate high blood pressure, many people have gone on low-sodium diets. They've listened closely to the National Academy of Sciences' advice that we should limit our sodium intake to 1,100 to 3,300 milligrams a day (one teaspoon of salt contains 2,000 milligrams). Given that most Americans ingest between 4,000 and 15,000 milligrams a day, mostly from food, that's a good idea, particularly if you are prone to high blood pressure.

If you are older and you don't have high blood pressure, congestive heart failure, or kidney problems, however, you should *not* overly restrict your salt intake, according to Dr. Michael Freedman, director of the Division of Geriatrics at New York University Medical Center. Dr. Freedman points out that aging kidneys have trouble conserving sodium, and if you add a salt-restricted diet to that problem, you can get into real trouble. Another problem for many older people is that when they stop using salt, they stop eating, which can lead to malnutrition.

When older people consume less than two grams of salt per day, they may get into real trouble. Salt deprivation can cause confusion or make older people go "crazy." Dr. Freedman told of recently getting a call regarding an eighty-six-year-old businessman who had just been admitted to the hospital. An active and vigorous person who still went to his office and to meetings every day, he had suddenly started acting bizarrely and became totally confused. The family had been told that he was probably demented and would have to be institutionalized. When Dr. Freedman went to see him, he found that the patient, who was on a salt-restricted diet, had also been put on diuretics. After assessing the situation, Dr. Freedman ''prescribed'' pickles and a corned beef-and-pastrami sandwich from the Second Avenue Deli. By the next morning, the patient was fine, all the ''craziness'' was gone, and he was able to go back to work.

Even when older people have hypertension, Dr. Freedman cautions, the recommendations regarding salt restriction don't always apply. Unlike hypertension in some younger people, hypertension in the elderly generally is not due to volume overload; it seems to have more to do with the blood vessels being less compliant. Because cardiac output is also lower, he says it's important not to deplete the volume or to further decrease cardiac output.

If your doctor recommends that you moderate your intake of salt, it's easy to do that simply by avoiding nuts, chips, crackers, pickles, and other salty items. In general, fast foods and processed foods, from soups to cheeses, contain large amounts of sodium. To determine the amount of sodium you're getting in various foods, look for the milligrams of sodium listed on the food label, or check the list of ingredients for sodium. Since ingredients are listed in order of their quantity, you'll know if the food is high in sodium if it's high on the list.

Caffeine

How many of you start your day with a cup of coffee, have a cola or a cup of hot chocolate during the day, and end up with a cup of tea in the evening? These popular beverages are not necessarily bad, but they do contain doses of caffeine, which is a drug that stimulates your central nervous system—which makes these drinks fundamentally different from water or fruit juice.

Doctors disagree on whether or not caffeine is dangerous. Some researchers say that people with heart trouble and high blood pressure should avoid caffeine altogether. They point to studies showing that from two to six cups of coffee can raise your blood pressure as well as produce profound effects on the electrical system of the heart, causing it to change rhythms. Coffee also stimulates an increase of adrenaline in the bloodstream, which may explain why large amounts of caffeine can create the symptoms of an anxiety attack— nervousness, irritability, restlessness, and insomnia.

If you have stomach problems, ulcers, or gastric irritation, you probably shouldn't be drinking coffee. Usually, caffeine promotes the secretion of acid in the stomach, which adds to your troubles.

If you're a tea drinker, you should be aware that you're receiving the same amount of caffeine from two cups of regular tea that you would get by drinking one cup of brewed coffee, or one and a half cups of instant coffee. A twelve-ounce bottle of cola contains approximately the same amount of caffeine as a cup of tea.

As for the positive benefits of caffeine, some recent studies have shown that older people experience good effects from two cups of coffee every morning. Coffee seemed to improve their mental alertness, make them feel more awake, and give them quicker reactions. Even investigators who generally don't advocate caffeine agree that a cup of coffee a day or small amounts of caffeine pose little risk to most people.

You probably know how your own system reacts to coffee or tea and can make your own choices about how much to drink. If you are tense or jittery, however, or if you have heart disease or trouble falling asleep, you should discuss the amount of caffeine you consume with your doctor. Remember not to use coffee, tea, or colas as your chief beverages. If your doctor tells you that you need to drink more liquids, she's not talking about coffee or leaf tea or herbal tea. She's talking about water or milk, or fruit and vegetable juices. Caffeine is a diuretic, and too much of it can contribute to your being dehydrated.

Herbal Teas

While most herbal teas don't contain caffeine, many of them contain chemicals that can affect you in harmful ways. If you're healthy and you enjoy herbal teas in moderate amounts, they probably won't cause you problems. But if you tend to have allergies, you should be aware—and beware—of the fact that many teas are made from any number of plants to which you could be allergic. You might choose an herbal tea with a wonderful and enticing name that combines several plants, one of which might be goldenrod, marigold, or chamomile. Those particular plants can cause allergic reactions if you're sensitive to ragweed or chrysanthemums. The severity of the reaction, like all allergic reactions, could be anything from mild to fatal. Substances in herbal teas can also interact with your medications, so be careful. Remember that drinking herbal tea is *not* like drinking water. Just as with coffee and ordinary tea, the substances in herbal teas are drugs. The difference is that you don't know all the drugs unless the company lists them on the product. Before making a purchase, read the list of ingredients on the box of tea. If there is not a complete list, don't buy it. If there is a complete list and you have any questions about it, check with your doctor, nurse, or pharmacist.

CIGARETTES—A HAZARD TO YOUR HEALTH

It's been well established that the use of cigarettes is the worst form of drug abuse in this culture and the greatest public-health problem in the country. Many studies have linked smoking to an increased risk of cardiovascular disease, including strokes and heart attacks. High blood pressure also increases the risk of heart and blood vessel disease, so the combination of hypertension and smoking increases the risk even more. As few as two cigarettes a day can increase your blood pressure. If you smoke *and* drink coffee, the blood pressure elevation is substantial and may last several hours. Besides being directly indicated as a cause of heart disease, bronchitis, emphysema, and lung cancer, smoking can have some negative interactions with your medicines. Smoking decreases the effectiveness of bronchodilators such as theophylline (Theo-Dur or Slo-Phyllin). It is also thought to decrease the effectiveness of benzodiazepines prescribed to reduce anxiety, such as Paxipam, Xanax, and Centrax.

While cigarette smoking is a preventable cause of death, it's not an easy habit to kick. Besides being a social addiction, it's one of the most powerful physical drug addictions around. According to Andrew Weil, M.D., at the University of Arizona College of Medicine, "the most flagrant example of drug pushing" can be seen in the tobacco industry. In an interview in *The Village Voice*, Dr. Weil said, "If you want to talk about death penalties for drug pushers, start with the executives of tobacco companies." Dr. Weil points out that while we may have some three hundred deaths a year from crack, there are something like three hundred thousand deaths from addiction to cigarettes, which the government continues to subsidize.

When you smoke, the nicotine rapidly rises in concentration and enters into the brain. Although it seems relatively harmless to the smoker, nicotine is a very strong drug. Researchers have found that nicotine is as addictive as amphetamines, cocaine, or heroin, and that for most people it is more addictive than alcohol.

ALCOHOL AND MEDICINE DON'T MIX

Some doctors believe that a glass of wine, or one to two ounces of alcohol a day, may actually be beneficial to health. In these moderate amounts, they say, it can reduce the risk of hypertension. However, consuming more than two ounces of alcohol a day has been found to lead to hypertension and other diseases.

Cocktail hour is such a sociable time that often we don't notice a growing dependency on drinks before dinner. And, at dinner, wine adds the "right touch" to a delectable meal—so much so that its side effects and addictive dangers are often ignored. With older people, alcohol can be particularly insidious. Blood alcohol levels are often elevated to the extent that they create or exacerbate disease states, but all too often this problem isn't recognized in the older person. If a younger person started stumbling around when he walked, was confused, or slurred his speech when he talked, we'd immediately suspect that he was drunk. If he had lost his memory or become malnourished, paranoid, or disoriented, we'd usually suspect alcoholism as a root cause. However, since the same symptoms in an older person can be caused by a variety of medical problems, and because they fit stereotypes of older people, these alcohol-related symptoms are often overlooked or mistaken for disease—making the incidence of alcoholism among the elderly much higher than most professionals imagine. It's only with careful investigation that physicians can sort out which declines are due to alcohol and which are due to real physical or mental problems that are independent of the drinking.

Chronic alcoholism is a common cause of vitamin B

deficiency, which may be associated with memory and cognitive defects. According to Dr. James Long, the use of other drugs combined with alcohol that are associated with (reversible) mental symptoms include the barbiturates and nonbarbiturate antianxiety agents, sedatives, and tranquilizers (such as Librium, diazepam, and glutethimide), non-narcotic analgesics (such as aspirin, Tylenol, and pentazocine), the salicylates, and narcotic analgesics. Often these drugs increase the intoxicating effects of the alcohol, and the alcohol reduces the effectiveness of the drugs and can interact with them to produce toxic effects. Other problems for older alcoholics include further vitamin deficiencies, dehydration, electrolyte imbalance, and depletion of carbohydrate supplies.

The aging alcoholic often doesn't get the treatment he or she needs. Family and friends don't intervene because sometimes they feel they'll be depriving an older person of pleasure or they assume the habit of drinking is too long-standing to change. Rather than encourage a friend or loved one to join Alcoholics Anonymous or to enter a detoxification program, they witness an inevitable decline.

"Nell Armstrong" was one friend who decided she had to take action on behalf of a loved one. Even though she hadn't realized that her companion was alcoholic, she learned that his deteriorating mental condition could be stopped, if not reversed, if he ceased drinking.

Nell's companion, "Melvin Thompkins," had been an architectural engineer in Baltimore, Maryland, until his retirement at sixty-five. He had been a social drinker all of his life. He only saw the doctor after Nell, his companion of eighteen years, insisted that he do so. During a vacation trip to Florida when he was sixty-eight, Melvin couldn't figure out whether to turn right or left when they drove out of the motel parking lot and forgot where he was going. On several occasions during and after the trip, he misplaced his glasses, his wallet, and other personal items. He seemed to have difficulty paying his bills—and Nell was worried.

When the doctor examined Melvin and gave him tests, she discovered a tremendous decline in his memory. Although neither Melvin nor Nell thought that he had a drinking problem, their social life revolved around cocktails with friends, wine with dinner, and drinks with bridge (brandy afterward). Nell had noticed that Melvin's memory problems were worse when he drank, and although he told the doctor he had cut down on alcohol, he continued to have wine with lunch, one drink before dinner, and wine or beer with dinner.

The doctor recommended that Melvin go into the hospital for detoxification and completely stop drinking. The dementia, she was quite sure, was induced by alcohol. Some of the damage most likely was permanent, but if he stopped drinking, his chances for living without further decline were good. She explained that it would take him longer to go through detoxification than it would a younger person because it would take longer to get the alcohol out of his system.

"Look at his day-to-day functions," she said to an interdisciplinary geriatric team of nurses, social workers, and other doctors with whom she was talking. "Melvin is an architectural engineer, yet he loses things in his apartment and can't remember which way to turn on the street. His functional deficits are profound for someone so well educated and smart! He and Nell both need to deal with his drinking. They also need to discuss dementia and how he wants to deal with a decline that is bound to continue if he keeps on drinking."

The Ravages of Alcoholism

When one out of five Americans reports that he has sought help either for himself or a family member because of alcoholism, it shouldn't surprise anyone that alcoholism is commonly found among the elderly. Approximately two-thirds of elderly alcoholics have been drinking heavily all their lives. Many of them have brain and liver damage due to their long history of drinking. The other third are called "late-onset" alcoholics. They are people trying to mask or cope with the death of a spouse, depression, or loss of work or income. Ironically, sometimes people drink out of despair over their poor health or multiple physiological problems. Late-onset alcoholism can develop within a few months or a year, while it usually takes five to fifteen years for alcoholism to develop in a younger person.

Modest Social Drinking

Even people who are only moderate drinkers can get into serious trouble when they combine their drinks with their medicines—whether those medicines are taken the day before, the same day, before, during, or after dinner.

Light drinkers, by the way, also receive more of an impact from alcohol as they age. Age decreases tolerance for alcohol in most people. As a result, the same amounts that you might safely have consumed when you were younger can have harmful effects in later life. Brain neurons are more sensitive to alcohol in advanced age, so drinking tends to more readily disturb your sleep and your sexual experiences. Not only does the aging central nervous system respond more sensitively to alcohol, but as the liver and kidney functions decline, more alcohol stays in your system for a longer time and has a more dramatic effect on you. Even without extreme consequences, the hazards are significant when they interact with the diseases of older people. Merely one drink can mask pain from angina and reduce its value as a warning sign. Because alcohol is carried by the bloodstream to all the organs, it can aggravate already existing diseases of the liver, pancreas, intestines, blood, and nervous system.

The effect of alcohol on the liver and on metabolism is what interferes with most medications. Since the detoxification process is usually much slower in the older body, the introduction of any new drug is likely to interact unfavorably with the alcohol in the body. As records from hospital emergency rooms show, it's not unusual for mixtures of drugs and alcohol to result in coma or death.

Drug and Alcohol Interactions
Dual dependence on drugs and alcohol often begins when a person is drinking excessively. Drinking adds to or stimulates irritability, anxiety, depression, and sleeplessness. If the physician (usually unaware of the drinking) prescribes tranquilizers to treat these symptoms, the patient can be thrown into a cycle of using the medicine and alcohol to counteract each other. The pills counteract the effects of drinking, and when the effect of the pills wears off, the person drinks to feel better and gets hooked on both. This syndrome can even happen to a moderate social drinker who is combining antidepressants with alcohol.

If you're taking Librium, Dalmane, Valium, or some other sedative or tranquilizer that slows down your central nervous system, you shouldn't be drinking alcohol at all. If you do, you're taking a risk with your health. Both the drugs and the alcohol are central nervous system depressants. They may feel good at first, but together they'll eventually depress your system severely. One of the biggest dangers from the combination of sedatives with alcohol is that people become much more accident-prone. An older person who has to get up in the night to go to the bathroom is much more likely to stumble and fall and risks broken bones as a result. Over-sedation is also particularly dangerous when it makes you drowsy and immobile. Drowsiness is not a side effect of sedative drugs; it's a *characteristic* of their use. They're supposed to make you feel that way.

Sometimes the combined effect of drugs and alcohol creates a much stronger drug effect than you would have without the alcohol. For instance, when you combine alcohol with pain relievers such as Percodan or sedatives like Nembutal, the synergistic effect can be quite dangerous.

When "Mabel Stevenson" began drinking, it never occurred to her that she would be over-sedating herself. She had taken sleeping pills for years, but when she started having a couple of cocktails in the evenings, she soon got into the habit of sitting around in her large red chair during the daytime as well. "I just seemed to be tired all the time," she reports. "And I didn't really care about anything. I started watching the soap operas, and then sometimes I'd realize I'd been sitting for hours. Walter Cronkite would come on with the evening news, and I'd still be in my bathrobe. Some days I didn't even feel like getting out of bed in the morning. I just felt miserable. If I hadn't gotten pneumonia, I suppose I would have just faded away and died lying there."

An alert and caring social worker who met Mrs. Stevenson in the hospital made her aware of what the combination of alcohol and sleeping pills was doing to her. The social worker directed Mrs. Stevenson to a nearby senior center when she left the hospital and saw her weekly for several months. Now Mrs. Stevenson drinks one glass of wine each evening and has sworn off the sleeping pills altogether.

She was lucky. Often chest infections like pneumonia are a terminal disease for the elderly. And ironically, simply the immobility of the older person—not a walk in the rain or a slosh through the snow—can lead to pneumonia. Over-sedation that causes immobility can adversely affect the cardiovascular, respiratory, gastrointestinal, and urinary systems.

Other combinations of medicines and alcohol are also disastrous. Similar complications can result from other over-the-counter medications. The combination of alcohol and over-the-counter sleeping pills, for instance, can decrease intellectual functioning. The combination

of alcohol with certain over-the-counter preparations, such
as Sudafed, can create delirium. Aspirin can throw you
for a loop. Toxic doses of aspirin alone can be similar to
alcohol intoxication, producing varying degrees of confusion, stupor, paranoia, or delirium. When aspirin is
combined with alcohol, the response can be extreme.

A Familiar Story

Like many older people, "Edna Godfred," the mother
of "Marie Laughten," eased into combining alcohol
with medications without realizing what she was doing.
The way she multiplied her troubles is a familiar story.

"After my younger sister graduated in 1968, my
mother and father moved to northern California," Marie says, trying to recall the earliest stages of her mother's problems. "My father had been a banker in a small
town in Oklahoma, where my mother raised seven children. She had taught school during the war, and she
was strongly opinionated. He was never ambitious, and
she was very ambitious. Their differences showed up as
they got older and their joint projects were over. Nevertheless, when he died in 1982 from acute leukemia,
my mother was lost. He'd always had the moral authority, and even though it hadn't seemed like it, her iden-
tity was wrapped up in being his wife and our mother.
Now she was isolated and lonely. She couldn't hear,
she had osteoporosis, and she felt totally lost. I was
noticing aberrations—she seemed to drop things a lot,
but the patterns didn't really hit me.

"Theoretically, she was very interested in her health
and was going from one doctor to another to find out
the *physical* reasons for her problem. She knew something was wrong, but she wanted to think the cause was
exclusively physical. She wouldn't acknowledge any
biochemical or emotional connection because she's
learned that it's *your own fault* if you have these problems. She feels there's shame in being ill, that you're
at *fault* if you're ill.

"Then last year, she had a transient stroke while she was playing bridge. She was taken to the emergency room. They operated on her carotid artery, and she physically recovered, but the doctor realized she was drinking and said she couldn't drink at all after this.

"It was the kind of problem you had to see up close for a while to know what was happening," says Marie. "When she moved in with my brother and his wife, they didn't notice at first. They have a big house with five kids and a lot of chaos. But then her behavior started to seem really strange, and it became clear that she was having mental problems. She'd have real rages and then appear to be in control again. Then she'd be depressed. I remember depression used to be defined as 'frozen anger,' and that seemed to fit. Emotionally, she was in terrible shape. Then she got Asian flu and went down to one hundred and two pounds from one hundred and thirty-two.

"Last year, we bought popular books on medication-induced depression. The doctor had put her on antidepressants in 1981. When I realized how much she was drinking, I wrote him a letter saying she was overmedicated on various tranquilizers and sedatives and was also abusing alcohol. I said I thought he should know that about her medicine and alcohol. He took her off some things and put her on an antidepressant. At the time she was on meprobamate, which she'd been on for years, and one hundred and sixty milligrams a day of Inderal.

"She'd kept various prescriptions going for years. We didn't realize it, but she had two pharmacies sending her tranquilizers on a regular basis. Then she added gin and later bourbon to the roster, plus she was eating less and less at the same time.

"She was also borderline diabetic. That was the physical thing. She was on medication for diabetes, but because she ate so little, it was too large a dose. They learned at the hospital that she had low blood sugar.

We learned from them that you have to control *every-thing*.

"They asked questions like, 'Is she tired in the morning?' Yes, she was! She'd been keeping the light on all night to keep from going crazy. She had to stay up all night to stave off the furies.

"Now we know that alcohol was self-medication. Afterward, she'd recall the pleasure and not the immediate aftereffects.

"Finally we got her into a health-related facility, one that accepted that she had mental and emotional problems along with her physical ones," says Marie. "We had a hard time getting her to go. It's a habit that you respect your mother and do what she says. It's hard for kids to say, 'No, you can't do that anymore; it's not good for you.' You're not used to saying no to your parent, but the psychiatrist told us, 'You have to be tough. She's strong, and you have to be strong.' Now they have her totally off alcohol, and she's on nortriptyline and a little bit of haloperidol [Haldol], which seem to be helping her."

A change of environment, getting her off multiple medications and alcohol, and treating her true underlying disease—depression—restored Edna Godfred's life. Like many people, she was using alcohol as an antidepressant, when being treated for depression was what she needed to stop drinking.

"Now she says she feels good, exactly like she did when she came in, but she can't remember how she really felt. She's gotten interested in other people and interested in clothes again," says Marie. "We think that a lot of why this happened was because she couldn't cope with aging and her loss of control over other people. Now she's beginning to live her own life again and to realize she's worthwhile in and of herself."

COMBINING FOLK CURES AND DRUGS

Beyond the "normal" use of salt, coffee, alcohol, and food, you may be in the practice of treating your symptoms of discomfort or illness with certain tried-and-true practices that seem to be non-pharmacological. For instance, when you feel a cold coming on, you may be a proponent of chicken soup or ginseng tea. You may eat large amounts of garlic or even chew willow bark if you're in pain. Many times the cures we have learned from our ethnic traditions work as well as anything else to relieve the discomforts of colds or limited illnesses that go away with time.

"A lot of people cure themselves of the symptoms of their colds by drinking herbal teas they make from goldenseal or comfrey," says geriatric nurse Sylvia McBurnie. "For many people, they work, but they can be a problem for people with allergies. People also have many other curative measures they use that are based on their own cultural or religious folklore. Many Hispanics, for instance, classify diseases as 'hot' or 'cold' and won't take prescriptions or follow special diets if they don't fit the definition of the heat or the coolness of the illness. Others believe that it's good to drink brandy for a cold, and they'll take their cold tablets with brandy in the morning and in the evening."

If you are using any home remedy or cure other than chicken soup, or if you are drinking alcohol or restricting your diet in any particular way to improve your condition, make sure that you let your physician know what you're doing. Even if you're only making a special tea, it still has an effect on your body and the potential to interact with a medicine that you're taking. Many folk drugs contain substances that are similar to the properties in medicines.

If you tell your doctor all the substances you're taking, he'll have a way to evaluate their potential interactions with your medications. Be wise and don't get yourself into a situation where you're the victim of adverse drug interactions.

CHAPTER 9

★

*Over-the-Counter Drugs—
Fads and Facts*

"In August 1980, I was anxious to lose ten pounds before my son's wedding, and seeing a large display of diet pills by the checkout counter at the drug store, I asked the manager if they worked; it seemed too good to be true. He said, 'A lot of my customers seem to get good results with Dexatrim.' After reading the warnings on the back and seeing I had none of the illnesses, such as high blood pressure, diabetes, or glaucoma, or any of the others listed, I thought it would be safe and bought the extra-strength size. I was on no other medication and, at sixty-one, was in excellent health.

"I took one pill a day, as directed, for nearly three months, went on a strict diet, and lost ten pounds. On November 17, 1980, I had a cerebral hemorrhage and nearly died. I spent eighteen days in New York Hospital. Since then, my memory and my hearing have deteriorated and my coordination is very poor. Worst of all, I have trouble with words, often saying "hot" when I mean "cold," or "house" when I mean "hotel." Sometimes whole sentences come out the wrong way.

"However, I feel I am one of the lucky ones, as I can still function fairly well on my own.

"Unfortunately, as long as these pills are readily

available, no amount of warnings will stop people from taking what seems like an easy way to lose weight. I have friends who, in spite of what happened to me, are still taking Dexatrim, confident it won't happen to them. These diet pills are dangerous and should be taken off the market.''

—*Statement of Anthea Sachs, testifying before the Subcommittee on Health and Long-Term Care of the U.S. House of Representative's Select Committee on Aging, July 21, 1983.*

One evening a couple of years ago, when my son Zachary was six years old, he came out of his bedroom rubbing his eyes. ''I can't get to sleep, Mom,'' he said. ''Could you give me some Nyquil?''

''What's Nyquil?'' I asked, startled.

''It unstuffs your head and makes you relax and go to sleep,'' he answered with an unusual inflection and melody in his voice. ''For better, more effective rest, use Nyquil! You wake up refreshed!''

It was only after his recital of the jingle that I realized he was responding to a television advertisement he'd heard.

''No, honey,'' I said, ''I won't give you Nyquil, but I'll give you a glass of milk. It will help you relax, and then you'll get right to sleep.''

When advertisements such as Nyquil's appeal even to a six-year-old who has no experience with such matters, it's not hard to imagine why older Americans are ready to spend hundreds of millions of dollars to alleviate congestion or a troubled night's sleep. Just like many other over-the-counter drugs (OTCs), Nyquil claims to treat multiple symptoms with multiple ingredients (''Five-Way Effectiveness''). It's billed as an antihistamine, analgesic, cough suppressant, and decongestant. Yet four of its active ingredients have been found to lack evidence of effectiveness, and its fifth ingredient is alcohol.

The practice of self-medication is common to all people who experience "self-treatable" health problems such as colds, skin problems, and minor aches and pains. According to the Nonprescription Drug Manufacturers Association, Americans spend $11.2 billion a year for some three hundred thousand over-the-counter remedies, not including vitamins and minerals.

According to consumer surveys by *Drug Topics* magazine in 1990, Americans spent $2.7 billion on cough, cold, and flu remedies; $5.8 billion on analgesics and digestives (which include laxatives, diarrhea remedies, sleeping aids, arthritis drugs, diet aids and vitamins); and $1.7 billion on external remedies (including eye drops, acne medications, external analgesics, and topical creams) purchased at retail stores.

WHY WE BUY OTCS

As you probably know, over-the-counter drugs (OTCs) are drugs you can buy *without* a doctor's prescription. We buy these products—from nasal sprays to cough medicines to cold remedies to sleeping tablets to weight-loss potions—mainly because:

- They're easy and we're uncomfortable. We want to feel better quickly, and it's faster to walk to the drugstore than to go to the doctor.
- We assume that the "problem" we're treating isn't serious enough to warrant a visit to the doctor.
- We think that if drugs are nonprescription, they're safe.
- They're less expensive, not only in terms of the drugs themselves, but because by medicating ourselves, we don't have to pay for a doctor's visit, a diagnosis, or lab work.

- We're convinced by TV advertisements that this medicine will cure our ailments.

Television ads, in particular, account for a large percentage of the purchases of over-the-counter products. Despite the fact that they affect our health and well-being, OTC medications are marketed on TV by the same methods as those used to promote laundry detergent, floor wax, shampoo, computers, and furniture.

Nevertheless, some observers think that the American public and older people in particular are not as gullible as it might seem. "People are getting smarter about their use of self-medications," says Mary Simons, assistant director of public affairs at the Proprietary Association. "It's a common assumption that older people buy more OTCs than any other people, but it's not true. If anything, they're cutting back and using them more cautiously."

According to surveys by the Proprietary Association and the American Association of Retired Persons (AARP), while older people use more prescription drugs than other age groups, this is not true of their consumption of over-the-counter products. In fact, older Americans use the same proportion of OTC products, or less, than middle-aged and younger populations. (The Proprietary Association found that teenagers and younger children are the biggest users of OTCs.) The House Subcommittee on Health and Long-Term Care reports that OTCs account for 40 percent of all the drugs older people use. While this still represents a larger number of purchases, it's not as high as has been assumed in the past. According to the surveys by the Proprietary Association and AARP, this more moderate use stems from the fact that while they have more chronic conditions, older people have fewer of the everyday complaints, such as skin problems or colds, for which people purchase OTCs. The OTCs older people do buy and put into their medicine cabinets most often are thought to be analgesics (painkillers), antacids, vitamins, and laxatives.

Their use of these drugs may be conservative when compared with their use of prescription drugs, but it's also important to ask what older people actually know about the over-the-counter remedies they do use.

HOW DO YOU CHOOSE?

Recently I thought about how little I know about OTC remedies as I walked through a large Thrift Rite drugstore looking for something to get rid of my cold symptoms. I counted seventy-eight cold, cough, and allergy preparations before I got bored and stopped counting. Then I walked by dozens of shelves lined with literally thousands of bottles and salves, capsules and tablets, before coming back to cold preparations. Compared with "the olden days," today's selection of "home remedies" is dizzying.

It used to be that medicines were peddled from the wagons of traveling medicine men or sold from the shelves of the local general store. When a mother was purchasing her stock of medicines, she had no labeled ingredients, patient information, or precautions to go by; she just took the word of her neighbor, the patent medicine peddler, or the storekeeper. Most of the family's problems—from fever to fungus to toothaches to worms—were treated from the same bottle of medicine. I wondered how anyone these days is supposed to choose among the thousands of products on pharmacy shelves. It seemed clear to me that I didn't have much more to go on than if I'd talked to a medicine peddler, who, I felt, might be almost as reliable as a television commercial, which lacks the personal touch and doesn't even have to pass this way again to hear the results of its recommendations.

When I finally picked a cold "remedy," I noticed

that I'd made my choice based on what I'd heard advertised. I realized that the $2 billion a year the pharmaceutical industry spends to promote its products is probably well worth it. People respond to those ads. I also realized that usually if I haven't chosen a product recommended by a doctor or a friend, I almost invariably choose an advertised brand over one with a name I don't recognize, even though I can see from the label that they have the same ingredients. Irrational as it may be, the brand name makes me feel safer. Obviously, this response is exactly what advertisers aim for.

According to a study by the Proprietary Association, my method is a common one. Most people using nonprescription drugs rely on information from advertisements and, to a much lesser extent, on information from package labels. Ads clearly aren't unbiased; they're designed to sell products. As for labels, they often do contain valuable information if you can read the print and interpret it. Usually, however, the print is too small to be able to read without a magnifying glass. This makes OTC labels almost impossible for most older people to read. And as for knowing which ingredients are safe and effective, that's no easy task either.

How can you find out the truth about any over-the-counter product? We've *heard* that Preparation H shrinks hemorrhoids, but does it really? Anacin is supposed to work faster than plain old unbuffered, store-brand aspirin. Is that true?

A STANDARD FOR JUDGING

Thirty years ago, we didn't have anything to go on in choosing our OTC products. Manufacturers didn't have to let us know the basis of the potions they used in their products, nor did they have to prove that their claims were true. In 1962, however, Congress revised the Food, Drug and Cosmetic Act and required that all new drugs, or old drugs claiming new uses, had to be effective as well as safe. (The original Food and Drug Act was passed by Congress in 1906. It called for protecting the public from hazardous foods, drugs, cosmetics, and medical devices.) Now, even though the law doesn't require prescriptions for the purchase of OTCs, it doesn't exempt their makers from the same prescription controls that are supposed to protect the public. These controls are considerable. For instance, the processes by which the OTCs are manufactured are subject to FDA inspection. In addition, labels must be truthful. They must list ingredients and include warnings that have been specified by the FDA. Recommended doses are supposed to be appropriate, and false claims are not allowed. Within these established constraints to protect the public, manufacturers are free to develop and market their own formulas.

In 1966, the FDA decided to remove unsafe and ineffective OTC drugs from the marketplace, but they didn't get started until 1972, when the FDA appointed national drug advisory panels to find out which products were safe and effective in compliance with the Food, Drug and Cosmetic (FDC) Act of 1962. Members of the panels included physicians, pharmacists, and other technically qualified people. By 1983, the FDA Advisory Panel, which consisted of seventeen national drug advisory panels, had reviewed more than seven hundred ingredients contained in approximately four hundred thousand products. They'd reviewed twenty-six therapeutic categories of drugs (such as products for coughs and colds, constipation, sleep, diarrhea, nausea, and vomiting). After eleven years of work, and twenty thousand volumes of information, these panels had found that *less than one-third of the over-the-counter products sold today could back up the therapeutic claims they made about their effectiveness*. They concluded that *70 percent of those ingredients were either ineffective or unsafe or that there weren't suffi-*

*cient data to allow the reviewers to come to any mean-
ingful conclusions on safety or effectiveness.*

As a result of the FDA Advisory Panel's reports to
date, many of the products found to have unsafe ingredients have been removed from pharmacy shelves. "If
they're not safe, they're not sold," says Mary Simons
of the Proprietary Association. "If their safety is questioned or studies show there may be some damage, then
the FDA orders them removed. They're very strict."
Others, like the Public Citizen Health Research Group,
disagree, saying that drugs that are unsafe, as well as
ineffective, are still on drugstore shelves.

It's true that despite dozens of reports from the drug
advisory panels, which are based on the 1962 law, drug
manufacturers still haven't been made to tow the line.
While the reviews of ingredients by the panels have
determined that some 70 percent of the ingredients are
not safe and effective, those determinations still haven't
been enforced by legal means, because the studies have
not been concluded, nor has the implementation process been set in motion. Although some companies have
voluntarily reformulated their products to leave out offending ingredients, others have not. Some of the ingredients are still being tested.

"It's a slow public process," said one doctor on the
FDA's OTC drug staff. "It's complicated, and no one
knows when we'll finish." When the review process is
completed and implementation gets under way—which
some pragmatists say won't be before the year 2000—
probably more products will be changed or removed
from shelves. This means that you and I are still purchasing—at an individual cost of *at least* forty dollars
a year—many over-the-counter products that have been
found ineffective.

To some observers, "ineffective" products are self-
limiting and don't pose major problems. "If products
aren't effective, people don't buy them," says Mary Simons at the Proprietary Association. "Effectiveness is

proven by purchase. If they don't work, people don't repurchase them, and the products don't survive.''

The Public Citizen Health Research Group says, however, that ineffective ingredients not only cost you additional money, but also expose you to the unneeded risks of swallowing ingredients that don't work. They point out that recovery is often attributed to ineffective OTCs because many of the products with multiple ingredients lacking evidence of effectiveness have at least one effective ingredient. Also, when an ineffective product does seem to make us feel better, it's because the problem for which we're taking an OTC is a ''self-limiting disease.'' In other words, it's a disease, like a cold, that gets better no matter what you do or don't do. So, if your symptoms respond quickly—faster than they would naturally—then it's probably because of that one ingredient (such as aspirin) in a multiple-ingredient pain-relief product.

HARD-TO-GET INFORMATION

In the meantime, it's difficult to find out on your own what's reliable and what's not when it comes to over-the-counter products. The FDA Advisory Panel doesn't put out a list of *products* that are effective or ineffective. It does put out a list of ingredients. That list, the ''Over-the-Counter Review of Ingredients,'' is approximately one hundred pages long. To get it, you have to apply through the Freedom of Information Staff.* Since these ingredients are not matched with products, that job is up to the consumer.

The Public Citizen Health Research Group has sifted through all these ingredients and matched them to prod-

*For more information, write to the Freedom of Information Staff, HFI-35, Food and Drug Administration, 5600 Fisher's Lane, Rockville, Maryland 20857.

ucts in their book, *Over-the-Counter Pills That Don't Work*. They say that many popular nonprescription drugs lack evidence of safety and effectiveness, and they recommend many effective, safe alternative treatments. Their comments regarding products containing ingredients reviewed by the national drug advisory panels named by the FDA are simple and straightforward. For instance, they say: Preparation H, which contains shark liver oil and live yeast cell derivative, does *not* shrink hemorrhoids. (Keeping the rectum clean and dry and applying petroleum jelly or zinc oxide is an effective alternative.) Anacin, which contains aspirin and caffeine, doesn't work any better for an ordinary headache than plain generic aspirin, plus you may have side effects from the caffeine. (For migraine headaches, however, aspirin with caffeine may actually work *better* than plain aspirin.) Listerine mouthwash does not kill germs on contact, nor have the ingredients of Robitussin cough syrup been proved effective.

A COMMON MISCONCEPTION

Somehow many of us have come to believe that if we can buy the medicine ourselves, if the doctor doesn't have to write a prescription for it, it's safe. Obviously, this isn't necessarily so.

Even the three out of every ten products that do provide effective therapeutic relief for the symptoms they claim to treat may not be safe for you to take—depending on your disease and the other medications you're taking. Many of these products can help you, but they're also powerful drugs in and of themselves. Some of them used to be prescription drugs—and are now sold without a prescription. Chlor-Trimeton, for instance, is now easy to get, whereas in the old days, you had to find a doctor for a prescription.

Just like prescription medications, over-the-counter

drugs have side effects. The chemicals in them can get you into trouble when they interact with food, alcohol, and other medications.

"People think OTCs are harmless," says Dr. Bruce Kimelblatt of the Department of Pharmacy at Mount Sinai Hospital, "but they're not. For instance, even small amounts of aspirin can cause bleeding. Antacids can reduce drug absorption and can reduce the effectiveness of digoxin. When you take an antacid with another medication, the altered effect can be offset by staggering the administration times."

Sometimes, patients don't think to tell their doctors that they're taking an antacid, aspirin, or a laxative—and run into complications when those OTCs interact with their regular medicines. Dr. Kimelblatt points out that a person who hasn't told his doctor which over-the-counter preparation he's taking may find himself in serious trouble as a result of interactions that could have been avoided. For example:

- Aspirin can increase the effect of blood thinners—a serious matter for people with peptic ulcer disease, who then are at risk for hemorrhage.
- Chronic use of aspirin can also lead to iron-deficiency anemia due to blood loss.
- Cough syrup that contains alcohol can interact disastrously with tranquilizers.
- Medicine with salt can increase your blood pressure.
- Sominex can aggravate glaucoma.

Even when OTCs are used under a doctor's supervision, patients sometimes get into serious trouble from them. Faith Smiley was lucky to live through her ordeal from aspirin. "I'd had a little heart attack," says the eighty-one-year-old retired teacher from Stanwood, Washington, "and the doctor said I should take several aspirin a day. I never thought about it. I was taking four or five five-grain tablets a day with water, but not with

food or anything. Then one day when we were going to
Seattle on the bus, I fainted. I didn't know it, but I was
bleeding internally.

"I got the bus driver to stop and I was running around
desperately looking for a phone," says her artist husband, Bruce Smiley. "I thought it was her heart, and I
was scared to death. Finally I got a policeman, who
called an ambulance to come pick her up. By then she
was throwing up quite a bit of blood."

To make matters worse, Faith's sister, Helen, a nurse
who was along on the bus, put a nitroglycerin tablet
under Faith's tongue.

"When she passed out like that, I thought it was her
heart," Helen said. "But I shouldn't have! It wasn't her
heart, and it wasn't good at all to give her the nitroglycerin. The nitroglycerin stimulates your heart and
makes it pump harder. That dilated the blood vessels
and just made her bleed more! Here she almost leaves
us, and I am adding to the problem by making her bleed
more. I've felt so terrible about that since it happened.
It really taught me a lesson."

The other medication Faith had been taking when she
began taking the aspirin was a prescription drug, Tolectin, a mild anti-inflammatory painkiller that she took
for bursitis. A serious adverse reaction to Tolectin is
intestinal bleeding, so, combined with aspirin, it had a
synergistic effect.

After the scare, the doctor took Faith off both the
Tolectin and the aspirin and treated the bleeding ulcers—
which had probably been caused by the medications—with
Tagamet.

Faith's situation points out, once again, how important it is never to share your medicines or assume that
someone else has the same problems you have. Your
intervention might help, but it might cause the other
person harm or result in a fatality.

Even small doses of aspirin can cause problems. Dr.
Alvin Ahern, eighty, was taking one-half of an aspirin

a day, under doctor's orders, as a blood thinner. When he started having frequent nosebleeds, he became anemic. Stopping the aspirin stopped the nosebleeds and the anemia. Now he takes one-eighth of an aspirin a day. Many times the "recommended dosage" is much too high for the older person. Just as doctors recommend that initial doses of prescription drugs should be small for older people, they also recommend starting with very small doses of OTCs. It's usually safe to use one-fourth of the "recommended dosage" for starters and build it up if needed.

DANGERS OF ASPIRIN

It's easy, if you have a headache, a fever, a backache, or a swollen ankle, just to reach for the bottle of aspirin. Taking an aspirin doesn't seem like a big deal. Millions of Americans take aspirin every day for a variety of reasons. It's something that works and has been working for years. For many years, doctors thought of aspirin as nontoxic, but now they know that it can have a powerful and sometimes quite harmful effect on the gastrointestinal tract. While it's very effective in relieving pain and reducing swelling, it's also irritating and corrosive in the stomach and causes some internal bleeding.

Ever since people have learned that aspirin can be used as a blood thinner, the rumor has spread that you should take an aspirin a day to keep from having a heart attack. Everybody who takes one aspirin anytime will have a little bit of bleeding. That's okay when you only have an aspirin every now and then. But if you take aspirin daily, without medical supervision, it can cause real problems. Long-term use, for instance, can lead to peptic ulcers. If you have ulcers or gastritis, you shouldn't take aspirin in any form.

Also, even if you had too much to drink and you want

to take an aspirin for your hangover, *don't* do it if you're taking certain other medications. Aspirin (acetylsalicylic acid or A.S.A.) is known to cause problems if combined with blood thinners, such as Coumadin, heparin, or Dicumarol; any oral diabetic medicine; any medication for gout; Corticosteroids, such as cortisol and prednisone; and Methotrexate, which is used in psoriasis and cancer therapy.

Remember the following tips on aspirin:

- Buffered aspirin hasn't been proved to be any "gentler" to the stomach than plain aspirin.
- Even ibuprofen, which is a good drug for people who can't tolerate aspirin, can be hard on the stomach if used regularly.
- To minimize stomach irritation, take aspirin with a full glass of milk or water or immediately following a meal.
- If you're taking aspirin, tell your doctor about it.
- Ask your doctor about sucralfale (Carafate) or a new drug called misoprostol (Cytotec), which helps prevent stomach damage from aspirin and nonsteroidal anti-inflammatory drugs.

COMBINED-INGREDIENT DRUGS

Over-the-counter drugs with combined ingredients pose particularly difficult problems. That's because in addition to the single ingredient that could alone be effective for your particular problem, one or more ingredients are thrown in to reach a wider audience with a wider array of symptoms. These ingredients are "fixed" in ratio to one another. In other words, the dosage of each ingredient is constant, and whether the drug is safe and effective depends on whether the ingredients taken *together* are safe and effective. Some products contain as many as five different ingredients—all of which are supposed to address different symptoms—and patients usually aren't aware of all the ingredients. Physicians, pharmacists, and technical people all agree that there's no evidence to prove that increasing the number of different ingredients in a medicine make it better or more effective. On the other hand, they point out, we *have plenty of evidence that the likelihood of unwanted side effects clearly increases proportionally with the number of drugs consumed.*

A large number of OTC products sold are combination medications. If you're pulling the bottle off the shelf, you might not think to wonder what ingredients a particular cough syrup contains. You probably think of it as a single product. But it may have two different drugs in it. One of those ingredients may be very harmful to you. For instance, if you can't take aspirin, you may not realize that Excedrin, Bufferin, and Alka-Seltzer all contain aspirin. If you took one of them, you could end up with a bleeding stomach because of the "hidden" components. The Public Citizen Health Research Group, in their book *Over-the-Counter Pills That Don't Work*, advises consumers *not* to take combination cold remedies for the following reasons:

• They contain antihistamines and/or oral decongestants; neither should be taken for the common cold. (They do relieve symptoms, but they don't make you get over the cold any faster.)
• They contain drug ingredients for the treatment of a wide range of symptoms. You probably don't have all the symptoms or don't have them all at the same time. The course of a cold is varied and unpredictable, and "shotgun" treatment doesn't help.
• Increasing the number of different drug ingredients is no assurance that the product will be more effective.
• Even when all the ingredients in a combination product are appropriate (which is not the case with any

cold products), the fixed ratio of ingredients makes these drugs a poor choice. It's very unlikely that every ingredient is present in a dosage that's correct for you. In an attempt to get enough of one ingredient, you may overdose on another.

Irrational Combinations

The advisory panels appointed by the FDA have found that many of the ingredients that were combined into one multiple-use drug, such as Nyquil, were "irrational" combinations that could not be proven to be effective. The National Academy of Sciences clearly came out against the use of combination drugs in an earlier report on whether over-the-counter drugs had the power to produce desired effects. "It is a basic principle of medical practice that more than one drug should be administered for the treatment of a given condition only if the physician is persuaded that there is substantial reason to believe that each drug will make a positive contribution to the effect he seeks," the National Academy of Sciences said in their 1969 report. "Risks of adverse drug reactions should not be multiplied unless there is an overriding benefit. Moreover, each drug should be given at the dose level that may be expected to make its optimal contribution to the total effect, taking into account the status of the individual patient and any synergistic or antagonistic effects that one drug may be known to have on the safety or efficacy of the other."

When "Annie Calame," who is sixty-one, visited her eighty-four-year-old mother in Florida recently, she learned the hard way about combination cold remedies. Like many people, her good intentions as a "helper" and "prescriber" for her mother were foolish and ill-advised.

"My mother was sneezing and coughing and she had a headache, which she *never* has," Annie said in an interview. "I gave her a Coricidin tablet. My sister and I pop that stuff like candy. It didn't occur to me that she shouldn't have it. I gave it to her in the morning to help her clear up the cold, and during the night she woke up and started to cry. She had gone to the bathroom, and all she said was, 'I'm bleeding.'

"It was three A.M. We immediately put her in the car and rushed her to the hospital. They kept her there overnight until the bleeding stopped and said to never, never give her anything with aspirin in it. Even though she has angina and arthritis, which could indicate a need for aspirin, she can't take it because of other medications she's on for these conditions."

It never occurred to Annie that Coricidin contained aspirin, let alone something called chlorpheniramine maleate, or she probably would have wondered whether her mother should have it. She just thought of Coricidin as something to take for a cold. According to the FDA Advisory Panel, antihistamines lack evidence of effectiveness in treating the symptoms of a common cold, so even the ingredient in Coricidin that was supposed to have given Annie's mother some relief wouldn't have made any difference.

COMMON SELF-REMEDIES

As consumers, we Americans mainly buy over-the-counter preparations to treat irritating symptoms or to make ourselves more comfortable. We probably wouldn't buy as many products as we do if we didn't have a lot of misconceptions about how our bodies are *supposed* to behave. Dr. Bruce Kimelblatt at Mount Sinai says that many older people use laxatives because they commonly believe they're supposed to have a bowel movement once a day. "It's simply not true," says Dr. Kimelblatt. "It's normal for some people to have three BMs a day, whereas for others it's perfectly normal to have one bowel movement every three days.

"People usually don't need a laxative at all. If they

eat a high-fiber diet, drink plenty of water, and increase their activity, their bowels should function perfectly normally.''

Taking laxatives can create a problem. For instance, if they cause you to have too much diarrhea, your electrolyte balance can be thrown off by losing sodium, potassium, chlorine, and too much essential body fluid. Also, using a laxative may not be appropriate. If you're suddenly constipated, it may be an obstruction such as a polyp or a tumor. If you take a laxative, you're taking potent stuff to move the bowels.

Cold and Cough Preparations

It's amazing to think that those of us who are trying to get rid of our colds, coughs, runny noses, sore throats, allergies, and asthma spend more than $1.64 billion on preparations we hope will provide relief when there are no medicines that can kill the viruses that cause colds. Colds, which are spread by hands more often than they're spread through the air, can only be cured by time.

While older individuals worry about complications when they do catch colds, older people in general get fewer colds than younger people. There are some two hundred cold viruses in circulation. But whenever anyone catches a cold, he or she develops an immunity to that particular cold virus. According to Maryann Napoli, associate director of the Center for Medical Consumers in New York City, that may be why children have three times as many colds as adults.

Sleep Remedies

There are many over-the-counter medications—such as Compōz, Nytol DPH, Excedrin P.M., Unisom, Quiet World, Sominex, and Sleep-Eze—that are supposed to help you sleep better. Doctors I talked with felt that older people simply should not take these medications.

Sleeping disorders, they say, can be dealt with in natural ways—without medication.

If you have developed sleeping problems in conjunction with medication you're taking, you should be aware that some sleeping problems are *caused* by certain prescription or nonprescription medications. If you're having trouble sleeping and are taking drugs that stimulate your central nervous system (such as Benzedrine and Dexedrine, cough and cold remedies, asthma medicines like theophylline, diet pills, or drugs like MAO inhibitors or thyroid preparations), they well may be the source of your sleep problems. If you suspect your medicine, talk to your doctor about it because he can adjust the dose or even change the medication.

If you suddenly develop sleeping problems *after* you've stopped taking a drug that sedates your central nervous system, your doctor can help with that, too. While you were on it—whether it was an antianxiety drug such as Valium, a major tranquilizer (antipsychotic) such as Mellaril, or a tricyclic antidepressant such as Elavil, Tofranil, or Sinequan—it helped you sleep. Getting off it may leave you sleepless. Most likely, this is a problem you can solve with something other than an OTC. Getting more exercise outdoors, relaxing, getting up at the same time every morning, cutting out your afternoon nap, drinking a glass of warm milk, or taking a hot bath before going to bed—one or more of these may be all you need to get into better sleep habits.

All the active ingredients currently marketed as OTC sleeping medications are antihistamines. According to the Public Citizen Health Research Group, these drugs have many side effects, including dizziness, mental confusion, feeling faint, loss of appetite, and drowsiness. They are hazardous for a large number of people, including those with asthma, glaucoma, or difficulty urinating due to enlargement of the prostate gland. Antihistamines can interact dangerously with other drugs,

especially depressants, sedatives, medications for seizures, and alcohol. If you take a larger-than-normal
dose in an effort "to make sure it works," you can run
into severe adverse reactions, especially if you take it
in conjunction with alcohol.

Vitamins

The merits of those small organic substances we call
vitamins or "nutritional supplements" are still a subject of controversy. If you are standing in the drugstore
trying to figure out whether you ought to be taking vitamin E and lecithin along with C and B_6, you are not
alone. There's no easy agreement when it comes to vitamins. How much calcium and how much vitamin A
do you need? Is excess C really sloughed off without
any harm? Can you overdose on vitamins? Do you need
them at all?

Vitamins, as you know, are organic substances present in minute amounts in natural food you eat. They're
essential to your normal metabolism. A lack of vitamins and minerals can cause deficiency diseases. Within
our bodies, vitamins assist in the processing of other
nutrients, and they also help in the formation of the
cells, hormones, and chemicals used in our nervous
systems. Some doctors may prescribe vitamins for you,
whereas others will say you don't need to take any.

"If you eat a balanced diet, you don't need vitamins," says Dr. Kimelblatt of Mount Sinai. "If you do
use vitamins, you don't need megadoses. Doses tend to
be way out of line. We take too much! Twenty milligrams of vitamin C per day is enough to cure scurvy,
yet we take five hundred milligrams or more!"

Dr. David T. Lowenthal, director of Clinical Pharmacology and professor of Geriatrics, Medicines, and
Pharmacology at Mount Sinai School of Medicine,
agrees. "More is not better," he says. "Vitamins are
not innocuous! There are reports of toxicity with A, B_6,
and D."

Dr. Lowenthal points out that vitamins fall into two categories—fat-soluble vitamins (A, K, E, and D), which are absorbed with the aid of fats that are in your diet or bile from your liver, and water-soluble vitamins (C and B), which don't need fats or bile to be absorbed and are usually not stored in your body. Fat-soluble vitamins are stored in the body, so they can build up to toxic levels if you take too much. If you take A, D, E, and K vitamins two or three times a week, for instance, or eat food that gives you those vitamins, you'll be able to maintain those vitamins in your system, and your body can draw on what it needs. Water-soluble vitamins, on the other hand, are either used up quickly or pass out of the body, so they need to be taken every day in order to meet your daily requirement.

What constitutes your appropriate daily requirements may differ dramatically depending on what medicines you're taking and what chronic disease you may have. As a nutritional supplement, you may need only sixty milligrams of vitamin C, for instance, whereas for the treatment of a particular problem a doctor may recommend as much as 500 milligrams a day. Some researchers say there's no strong evidence to support the use of vitamin C in well-nourished people. While 100 to 150 milligrams of vitamin C can be absorbed by body tissues daily, they say the rest simply passes out of the body with the urine. Many people, however, swear by vitamin C. Nobel Prize–winner Linus Pauling, author of *Vitamin C and the Common Cold*, says he takes 18,000 milligrams of vitamin C a day and steps it up to 60,000 milligrams a day to ward off a cold when he feels one coming on. Some research shows that large doses of this vitamin do seem to shorten the duration of the common cold, but it hasn't been proven that it actually prevents colds. There's also some evidence that vitamin C may enhance the healing of wounds after surgery. Nevertheless, many doctors say that megadoses taken on a regular basis can lead to diarrhea, urinary tract infections, kidney and bladder stones, or an increased tendency of the blood to clot.

The FDA Committee on the Recommended Dietary Allowances states, "When a nutrient is used in excess of the RDA, or used to treat a disease that is not caused by an inadequate intake of that nutrient, the use is no longer nutritional. It is pharmaceutical. The nutrient is being used as a drug." Like other drugs, vitamins taken in massive quantities are considered overdoses.

Some risks that may be posed by megadoses of vitamins include:

- Overdoses of vitamin E may trigger headaches, blurred vision, cramps, nausea, fatigue, and muscle weakness.
- Too much vitamin A may cause headaches, symptoms of mental illness, weakness, liver damage, dryness of the skin, rashes, insomnia, nausea, diarrhea, joint pain, blurred vision, and hair loss.
- Vitamin D taken in megadoses may cause calcium deposits throughout the body, loss of appetite or nausea, kidney stones, high blood pressure, or high blood cholesterol.

Dr. Kimelblatt says that although studies haven't shown real harm from a normal intake of vitamin supplements, there's a great deal of misinformation about the use and effects of vitamins. "Vitamins cannot give you more energy," he says. "The FDA is requiring Stresstabs to revise their advertising since Stresstabs don't reduce fatigue or reverse symptoms of stress."

Vitamins can also interact with your other medicines. Dr. Kimelblatt warns that, for instance:

- Vitamin B_6 should not be taken in conjunction with the anti-parkinsonian medication L-dopa because the vitamin B_6 increases the breakdown of L-dopa before it gets to the central nervous system and thus blocks absorption.

Because of the potential complications involved, it's very important that you tell your doctor what vitamins you take. He needs to know every medication that you're on, including your over-the-counter vitamins.

WHAT SHOULD YOU DO ABOUT VITAMINS?

According to Dr. Jeffrey Blumberg, assistant director of the USDA Human Nutrition Center on Aging at Tufts University, the government sets the Recommended Daily Allowance (RDA) of vitamins at a level sufficient to prevent deficiencies and ups that slightly to cover the needs of 97 percent of the population.

"These requirements are sufficient to prevent deficiencies," he says, "but they're not necessarily what's required for optimal health."

As a general rule of thumb, Dr. Blumberg recommends that people take a daily nutritional supplement that's formulated at one times the RDA. (For more on RDAs for people sixty-five and up, see page 268 in chapter 11.) Even though this amount, when added to a healthy diet, may double the RDA, it provides a sufficient amount of micronutrients.

You cannot, however, buy just any one-a-day vitamin and assume that it will give you the proper proportions of vitamins you need. *You have to read the label on a multivitamin tablet and make sure that the amounts of vitamins in each table conform to the recommended daily allowance.* Many are not formulated to fit the required daily amounts. Some contain four or five times the amount of required vitamin C and E, while others contain only 2 percent of the requirement. "Some one-a-day vitamins are formulated in crazy ways," says Dr. Blumberg. "Some manufacturers try to get in every vitamin and mineral, but in order to make the pill a size and shape that can be easily consumed, they put in too little of everything. It makes no sense at all to take a supplement that provides only 5 percent of the RDA. Others are formulated with too much of two or three vitamins and not nearly enough of others. There are nutritional supplements formulated according to the RDAs, and those are the ones that people should use.''

According to Dr. Blumberg, nobody should take megadoses of vitamins. If you take ten times the RDA added to your diet, he says, then you're talking about a threshold of risk—particularly with vitamins D and A and selenium. ''There are very few justifications for megadoses,'' he says, ''and when there are, they're for therapeutic concerns, to make up deficiencies caused by burns, or particular diseases or malnutrition, and are prescribed under a doctor's supervision.''

When you're selecting a one-a-day vitamin, remember to read the label carefully to see what percentage of the U.S. RDA the vitamins contain. According to the Council for Responsible Nutrition, a trade association representing the manufacturers of nutritional supplements, the label should name the nutrient, its quantity in metric units, and the percentage of the RDA that represents. A good reference is *Recommended Dietary Allowances*, available from the National Academy of Sciences Bookstore, 2000 Wisconsin Ave., N.W., Room 384, Building 2, Washington, D.C.

ADVANTAGES OF SELF-MEDICATION

Even though there are dangers involved with certain ingredients of OTCs, there can be real advantages to self-medication. When the treatment is appropriate, it relieves the health-care system of a large workload of minor health problems. In addition, it saves you time and money and gives you a sense of responsibility and competence in managing your own health care. On the other hand, if you diagnose yourself wrong, you risk having a serious condition get worse before it's properly treated. Also, you risk adverse side effects from drug misuse or interactions that aren't being monitored by your doctor or pharmacist. Remember, too, that only one-third of the products you can buy have ingredients considered effective by the FDA. Are you sure you want to spend your money on products that may not be helpful?

If you take into consideration the possibilities involved in taking any nonprescription drug, you're likely to be careful and stay out of trouble. Cautious use can make all the difference in your safe management of OTCs.

TIPS TO REMEMBER IF YOU BUY ANY OVER-THE-COUNTER PREPARATION:

1. Are you buying this product for a minor and short-term problem? If you have a severe, persistent headache, frequently recurring indigestion, or other recurring pains, don't purchase an OTC. See a doctor for definitive diagnosis and treatment.
2. Buy your OTCs at your pharmacy, not at a grocery store or large all-purpose store that has no pharmacist.
3. Look at the package instructions. Read the label and the warnings carefully. Does this medicine contain more than one ingredient? Do you need more than one ingredient? Are you allergic to any of these ingredients?
4. Be particularly careful of medicines if they contain alcohol, antihistamine, aspirin, a decongestant, potassium, salt (sodium), or sugar.

5. Be particularly careful if you already take medicine for arthritis, diabetes, glaucoma, heart disease, high blood pressure, kidney disease, nervous conditions, or sleep problems.

6. Be careful if you have certain medical conditions such as gout, prostate problems, or ulcers.

7. Consult the pharmacist before you purchase any OTC. Ask him for help in making the best selection for your problem.

8. Tell the pharmacist all the medicines you're taking, both prescription and nonprescription. Ask him about any potential drug-interactions.

9. Ask the pharmacist about the dosage. In most cases, you'd be well advised to start with a reduced amount of the recommended dosage. For example, if the label recommends, "One to two tablets every four hours," don't start with two tablets. Start with one-fourth or one-half tablet and see what happens during the first four hours. Two is *not* better than one.

10. Don't leave the pharmacy without understanding how to take the medicine. How many times a day should you take it? Do you take it with meals, before meals, or after meals? Are there any foods or beverages you should avoid while taking this medicine?

11. Ask your pharmacist if there are any side effects you should watch out for with this OTC.

12. Don't use any OTC for more than a week. OTCs should be used only in treating minor or short-term, self-limiting conditions. A headache, for instance, should be alleviated

within a few hours, and a cold should be over within a few days.

13. *Always* tell your doctor about the nonprescription drugs, including vitamins, that you are taking. Bring all of them in for him to look at. Whenever you use an OTC on a long-term basis to manage certain problems (such as the use of aspirin in controlling arthritic pain or antacid for peptic ulcers), your doctor should always supervise its use.

Thanks go to The Parke-Davis Center for the Education of the Elderly, and Elder-Health Program at the University of Maryland School of Pharmacy for most of these suggestions.

THE 1, 2, 3's of OTCS*

1. Drink *one* full glass of water (eight ounces) when taking all medicines.
2. Antacids and laxatives should always be taken *two* hours before or after taking any other medicine, unless otherwise directed by your doctor.
3. Bottles of liquid medicine should be shaken at least *three* times before use.
4. OTCs are for short-term use. If your condition lasts more than *four* days, contact your doctor.
5. Read the *five* essential parts of the OTC label:
   - INDICATIONS: what it is used for
   - DIRECTIONS: how to take the medicine
   - CONTENTS: active ingredients and inactive ingredients
   - WARNINGS: side effects and drug interactions
   - PRECAUTIONS: precautions for use.

*Reprinted with permission from "OTCs Over-the-Counter Medicines," a pamphlet published by the Parke-Davis Center for the Education of the Elderly, and Elder-Health Program, University of Maryland School of Pharmacy, 20 North Pine Street, Baltimore, Maryland, 21201.

CHAPTER 10

Your Sexuality and Medication

"As long as one can admire and love, then one is
young forever. . . ."

—PABLO CASALS

"Some things are better than sex, and some things
are worse, but there's nothing exactly like it."

—W. C. FIELDS

"Nothing stops the sexual fantasies," says eighty-two-
year-old "Walter Moore" of Englewood, New Jersey.
"You don't perform sexually like you did when you
were twenty-two years old, but then, who does? Even
when I was thirty-eight, I looked back fondly on the
drive of those early days. Sometimes I think it'd be great
to have that kind of energy again, even for an afternoon.
Imagine having that stamina! But then I think, if everything else had to be the same again, it wouldn't be worth
it."

A retired research scientist and college professor,
Walter Moore is a trim and attractive white-haired man
who checks out four to five books a week from the
public library. He subscribes to *The New Yorker*, *Play-
boy*, *The Atlantic Monthly*, and *The New York Times*.
Every morning and evening he takes a walk with his
wife "Anna." Together they plant a large vegetable

garden each spring, maintain a lively exchange with their four children (and fourteen grandchildren), and are active in a nearby community church. Like other men his age, Walter has "slowed down a little" sexually since he was in his seventies, but still has a comfortable and very satisfying sexual relationship with his wife of nearly sixty-one years.

"I'd say that now we're probably more sensual than sexual in some ways," he said, "but we can still get the blood stirred up pretty good! Sometimes when I look at Anna, all those strong shimmies for her shiver through me like they always did. I think we'd both agree that it's not very different than it ever was, except that we have more time without interruption than we used to have. She says for her it's just gotten better and better. Don't tell her I said this, but she jokes that 'practice makes perfect,' and Lord knows we've had plenty of practice! There've been ups and downs for us, but these years are good ones. I think we're both pretty blessed."

Later, as Anna shelled peas and talked about her life with Walter, she told me, "We did have a setback at one point when they put Walter on a hypertensive [medicine] that really bothered him." She stared off into the distance and then shook her head, remembering. "That was a terrible time. I thought I was unattractive to him, and he thought he was getting old and falling apart. We were both pretty upset. We finally talked to his doctor about it, and he changed the medication. Then, like magic, things got normal again between us. Since then we've changed to a low-sodium diet, and now he doesn't really need any medication."

Walter and Anna Moore's active sexual life isn't uncommon for healthy couples in their seventies, eighties, and nineties. If their health is good, if they have a healthy sexual partner, and if they enjoy sexual activity, older men and women most likely will maintain an active sex life. Although grown children sometimes have trouble accepting that their parents are human beings with normal sexual desires and fantasies, and older people themselves sometimes feel that they "shouldn't be behaving this way," they don't lose their capacity or their need for that intimate and fulfilling contact.

LAYING THE MYTHS TO REST

Despite a great deal of evidence to the contrary, many people still believe the myth that older folks no longer have an interest in sex—and that besides that, they also lose their capacity. This simply is not the case. Studies have shown that *sexual activity may decrease slightly with age, but neither ability nor desire nor activity vanishes*.

In their pioneering and monumental work, *Sexual Behavior in the Human Male*, published in 1948, Alfred Kinsey, Wardell B. Pomeroy, and Clyde E. Martin established the fact that more than two out of three men over seventy were still sexually active. In subsequent studies of women, Kinsey noted that women reach their peak sexually in their late twenties or thirties and remain at that plateau through their sixties. Only after seventy, he said, would women show a slight decline in sexual response.

Researchers William Masters and Virginia Johnson, in their more recent studies of sexual behavior in older men and women at their Reproductive Biology Research Foundation in St. Louis, have noted that "human sexual response may be slowed by the aging process, but it certainly is not terminated." Their interviews with older people as well as their clinical testing of the aging body's physical reactions established in detail that the capacity for the cycle of sexual excitement, including plateau, orgasm, and resolution, is maintained throughout life.

In 1981, *The Starr-Weiner Report on Sex and Sexuality in the Mature Years* presented the results of a

survey of eight hundred people between the ages of sixty
and ninety-one and concluded that sex is a crucial part
of life for older people. The people surveyed expressed
a vital interest in their sexuality and said that their sexual experiences were just as gratifying now as when
they were younger.

The Starr-Weiner Report also established that:

- Sex gives older people a positive sense of well-being;
  it makes them feel beautiful, desirable, and exhila-
  rated.
- About 80 percent of people sixty-five and older are
  sexually active. Ninety-nine percent of the respondents said they desired sexual relationships.
- Nearly three-fourths said that sex is the same now
  as it was when they were younger; more than a third
  said it was *better* than when they were younger.
- Contrary to previous reports, there doesn't seem to
  be a decline in frequency of intercourse. Sexual frequency tends to remain consistent when a sexual
  partner is available.
- Reduced frequency, when it does occur, doesn't
  necessarily mean less pleasure. As one sixty-nine-
  year-old wrote: ''Sex is much more enjoyable and
  satisfying now. It used to be more frequent, but
  [now] each time lasts longer and has much greater
  sensory impact during climax for both of us.''
- Eighty-two percent of the survey responded that it
  was okay for older people to masturbate to relieve
  sexual tensions. Although they accepted masturba-
  tion in principle, only 44 percent of the men and 47
  percent of the women admitted that they themselves
  masturbated.
- The need to be touched, stroked, cuddled, and ca-
  ressed is a lifelong need. Physical contact in the sixties, seventies, eighties, and nineties is as powerful
  as it is during infancy, childhood, and early adulthood.

* * *

Doctors tell us that the main factors responsible for any loss of sexual desire or responsiveness in older people are:
* Fatigue—either mental or physical
* Overindulgence in liquor
* Depression or despondency
* Medications that have a negative impact on sexual function
* Loss of one's mate due to death or divorce
* One partner's withdrawal from sexual activity
* Undiagnosed diabetes, arteriosclerosis, cancer, or heart disease

"If a woman comes in to me and complains about a loss of libido, I know it's a symptom of depression unless she has a terrible disease such as heart disease, diabetes, or cancer," says obstetrician-gynecologist Dr. Gideon Panter in New York City. "Other than that, there's no minor condition or legal drug that makes a woman lose her libido. Usually if she's lost her libido and doesn't have a terrible disease, I refer her to a psychiatrist. Sex should be great for women. . . . If a woman stays alive long enough and has a sexual partner, her libido isn't going to stop."

"If a man is in otherwise good health," says gerontologist Myrna Lewis, coauthor of *Sex After Sixty* and *Sex After Forty*, "he is not likely to develop impotence that is physically caused. Physically based impotence is not a normal part of the aging process. It's connected with disease—and for a number of diseases, it can be one of the first symptoms. For instance, impotence is a symptom of undiagnosed diabetes and arteriosclerosis." There is psychologically based impotence as well. Often this is caused by severe depression or other factors that can be addressed by psychotherapy or work with a sex therapist.

A LIFETIME HABIT

Assuming that you are not afflicted by depression or disease, research shows that one of the most important criteria for whether you're interested in sexual activity in your older years is your level of interest and activity when you were younger. Some people have little interest in sex whether they're young or old. To them sex does not hold that much importance or doesn't seem central to their experience. According to Ms. Lewis, some people lose interest in sex as they get older because they're bored with the relationship they're in. It's no longer stimulating for them, and they haven't learned how to reinvigorate it. For others it may be that they had a great marriage but lost interest in sex after their spouse died. With some, a loss of interest in sex may have to do with work-related or retirement-related stresses or with religious beliefs. They may feel that a critical piece of sexuality is procreation, and so after menopause it's no longer appropriate. For the most part, however, people with high sexual energy and activity in their early years are far more likely to remain sexually active in their later years—which seems to be the case with many other activities and capabilities of older age as well.

"For a small but interesting group of people, sexuality becomes better as they grow older," says Ms. Lewis. "They've developed their personalities and they're more interested in others and more interesting to others. Or they may have had medical problems in their middle years—like prostate problems or problems around menstruation and menopause—that have been cleared up. Those people have fun and enjoy this new stage."

The moral of this story is that if you're someone who has always been interested in sex, you aren't necessarily going to suddenly lose that interest at the age of seventy-six or seventy-eight or even eighty-four. If for some reason you do, then you should look at your life circumstances, not your age. No matter what age you are, if you're under a great deal of stress or if you're depressed, your libido may suffer. If you don't like your spouse or he or she has died, that's another valid factor. Another possibility is that you're sick and you should see your doctor. If, however, you suddenly lose interest in sex and you're *not* depressed and you're *not* ill, your next suspicion should be medication.

THE SUSPECT MEDICATIONS

Many medications can cause sexual side effects. (See the list of drugs and their side effects on pages 252–3.)

Any medications that affect the central nervous system can have an effect on your sexual function, no matter how old you are. Severe anxiety states and depression, which many of these drugs are used for, often affect the libido—the psychic and emotional energy associated with your sexual drive. If you're given an antidepressant, you shouldn't automatically assume it will affect your sexual desire or performance in a negative way. Remember that loss of sex drive is one of the first symptoms of depression, and should always be considered. Geriatric psychiatrist Dr. William Gershell points out that, for some individuals, medications aimed at controlling anxiety and depression may foster a return of interest in sexual activity, depending on the person's normal level of sexual interest.

In other individuals, however, some antidepressants and some cardiac drugs and antihypertensive drugs can potentially interfere with sexual function by influencing the nervous system reactions that control the erection process in men and the mechanism for orgasm in women. Sleeping pills or sedatives can also affect the central nervous system and reduce sexual energy. According to Dr. Gershell, how a drug affects the individual is not entirely predictable. Some men on cardiac drugs, for instance, cannot have an erection; others simply experience reduced libido; still others find it difficult to reach orgasm.

Certain combinations of drugs can have more or less of an impact on your sexual feelings and experiences. You may need to work with your doctor to find the medicine or combination of medicines that best treats your condition and doesn't interfere with your sex life.

PHYSICAL CHANGES IN WOMEN

As a woman ages, it's normal for her vaginal tissues to take longer to become lubricated. Additionally, even when she's fully excited, there's often an insufficient amount of lubrication. Vaginal lubrication, as you may know, is produced by the congestion of the blood vessels in the vaginal walls. Physiologically, it's equivalent to the male erection.

Over the years, the vagina itself undergoes a reduction in length and width, and the walls get thinner. These changes can be traced to the decline of female hormones, such as estrogen, following menopause. The number of female sex hormones in a woman's body after menopause usually causes the tissues lining the vaginal walls to change both in flexibility and pliability. As you get older, there's less fatty tissue in the external genitalia; sometimes the labia shrink. There doesn't seem to be any change in the clitoris, which remains the main center of sexual stimulation. Excitement generated by clitoral stimulation seems to be the same in older women as it is in younger women. While a woman's responses may be slightly slower in older age, Masters and Johnson have established that a woman of eighty has the same potential for orgasm that she did at twenty.

Sometimes older women run into problems, however,

because the lack of lubrication and the thinning walls of the vagina (nerve endings are now closer to the surface) can make intercourse painful and cause a burning sensation.

There's no reason for you to accept pain or discomfort from intercourse. Don't assume that you must either avoid intercourse or get used to the discomfort "just because of age." Water-soluble (oil-free) vaginal lubricants, such as K-Y Lubricating Jelly, Ortho Personal Lubricant, Lubrin Vaginal Lubricating Inserts, and Lubafax, a vaginal suppository, as well as pure ointments like Vaseline, can be used before intercourse, and can also be used at other times to reduce irritation and dryness in the vagina.

Estrogen therapy is also an effective remedy for this condition. Estrogen can be applied topically or taken orally. Although there has been a great deal of anxiety and controversy over the use of oral estrogen, it now appears that its monitored use can be a health benefit. When research came out in 1975 that linked estrogen with a significantly increased risk of developing endrometrial cancer (the endometrium is the inner lining of the uterus), many women stopped taking estrogen. Recent studies suggest, however, that the cancer risk is dramatically reduced by new methods of administering estrogen that are safer than methods used in the past. Data linking estrogen with cancer were based on studies of patients who took estrogen alone, without progestin. Doses of estrogen given today are much lower than they used to be, and hormone therapy is now almost always given in combination with progestin, which greatly reduces and, according to some researchers, very probably eliminates the risk of estrogen-caused cancer. Many doctors, but not all, agree that if a woman takes estrogen with progestin on a cyclical basis, the cancer incidence is close to zero. Nevertheless many women choose not to take estrogen because of the cancer risk, and because there's also the possibility that estrogen use could be linked with gallbladder disease, breast cancer, and hypertension. In fact, studies indicate that only 10 percent of post-menopausal women currently receive estrogen replacement therapy.

Recent studies show that in spite of the risks, however, women on estrogen have longer life expectancy than women *not* on estrogen. The oral estrogen that's given in combination with progestin is taken in cyclical fashion, with a rest period of between five and seven days every month, which corresponds to a menstrual cycle, where a woman drops her estrogen production to almost zero. Research now indicates that this combination therapy protects against breast cancer, heart disease, and bone loss.

Topical Estrogen

"Jane Martin," a sixty-seven-year-old who's been married to her seventy-one-year-old husband for forty years, recently decided to ask her gynecologist about some changes in her sex life. "I felt really embarrassed," she said later, "but I had to talk to him about it. I told him our sex life isn't the way it used to be, but my husband and I still feel like doing it once a week.

"He said, 'That's fine! You shouldn't feel embarrassed about that. It's wonderful and normal that you're having sex at your age. There isn't any reason why you shouldn't enjoy it for many years to come.'

"I said that the problem is, my vagina burns when we do it. When he examined me, he said I had atrophic vaginitis. It was burning that way because the walls of my vagina were getting thin due to lack of estrogen. He said that the skin gets sensitive because the blood vessels shrink."

Mrs. Martin's gynecologist put her on estrogen, which she applies as a cream to the inside of her vagina on a regular basis. (An alternative would have been taking estrogen by mouth.)

Within three weeks, the burning sensation was gone, Mrs. Martin says, and it's never bothered her since.

Oral Estrogen

Dr. Panter tells about eighty-three-year-old "Mrs. Smith," whom he described as "charming, attractive, and vibrant," who came into his office and said, "Quite frankly, I want you to know I'm sexually active." Dr. Panter asked her if she had a lover, and she answered, "I have three lovers. One lives in New York, one in Paris, and one in Chicago." The woman's lovers ranged in age from seventy-one to eighty-five, and none of them knew about the others.

" 'I don't care what you find when you examine me,' " Dr. Panter reports Mrs. Smith saying. " 'I want to keep taking my estrogen. I don't want to lose my sexuality or my feelings. My system has been working all these years, and I know I've had such a good time because I've been on cyclic estrogen for the past forty years.' "

Although there's no medical evidence that estrogen increases libido or sexual performance, Mrs. Smith felt that estrogen had kept her in shape sexually.

"Some people never use estrogen and are perfectly fine," says Dr. Panter, "but others, such as Mrs. Smith, thrive on it."

Dual Purpose of Estrogen

Another reason some doctors recommend estrogen is that it's the only drug therapy that has proved effective in the prevention of bone loss. Currently one out of four women over the age of forty-five develops osteoporosis, a disease that results in vertebral crush fractures, broken bones, and a bent back that's commonly referred to as "dowager's hump." If you start taking estrogen orally at the age of fifty or at menopause, and if you maintain it, *you can prevent bone loss entirely*. If you begin to take estrogen at the age of sixty or seventy, after osteoporosis is already a problem, estrogen may prevent you from losing more bone calcium, but it won't reverse the damage that has been done or make you straighter.

Dr. Jean Coope, author of *The Menopause*, reports that women on long-term hormonal replacement therapy are 50 to 60 percent less likely to suffer fractures of the hip and forearm than women who do not take the hormones. Other doctors point out that osteoporosis indirectly causes the deaths of some thirty thousand women every year, which is at least eight to ten times the number of deaths from endometrial cancer. An analysis of the risks and benefits of estrogen replacement therapy by Dr. Brian Henderson at the University of Southern California indicates that it can result in a 41 percent saving in the lives of postmenopausal women.

"The doctor treating the patient has to balance the risks of osteoporosis with the risks of estrogen that can be cancer causing," says Dr. Diane Meier, assistant professor at Mount Sinai Medical Center and the chief of the Coffey Geriatric Clinic. "The doctor has to decide what's going to cause the greater risk. But women need adequate calcium in their diet and supplements if they don't get enough nutritionally. Also, they need to have adequate weight-bearing exercise [walking is one of the best]. Usually one multiple vitamin a day provides adequate vitamin D."

"Osteoporosis is an emotionally distressing disease," says Dr. Meier, who's directing a research program on osteoporosis, "and it's also physically distressing for most people. Some patients have no pain and discomfort, but many more have back and neck pain, abdominal pressure, and a body that's out of balance, which puts them at risk of falling. Their body mechanics are also off balance, so they have bowel irregularity and gas. They get aches and pains from walking around in an unnatural position.

"It's more than looking old and crippled. It's going from being a healthy and vital-looking sixty-five-year-old to looking ninety years old because of the compression of bones. It leads to a tremendous loss of body image and self-concept that in turn leads to a remarkable amount of depression. The depression is often so deep that patients lose interest in their work and their friends. They don't socialize and they don't exercise—which they need to do."

"A dowager's hump is the scarlet letter of old age," said another specialist who asked not to be quoted by name. "Our society doesn't give a lot of support to women who look old, and these women do look old. There isn't any more destructive visual symbol of aging. They feel they can't go out without being seen as decrepit. It does terrible things to their sense of themselves sexually. If they're widowed, their chances of pursuing a new relationship are dramatically inhibited by their own sense of being an undesirable woman."

"They say, 'I feel fine until I look in the mirror,' " says Dr. Meier. "Usually it's the last straw in a series of blows dealt out to older women. It's the final assault of having one's body look old and crippled."

Side Effects of Hormones

In their excellent book, *Menopause: A Guide for Women and the Men Who Love Them*, Winnifred Berg Cutler, Celso-Ramon Garcia, and David A. Edwards say that women who take estrogen don't usually experience any discomfort unless the dose is too high. If the dose is too high, you may have breast tenderness, more vaginal discharge due to large increases in cervical secretions, weight increase, leg cramps, fluid retention, headaches, or unscheduled uterine bleedings. These symptoms of overdose, they say, can continue for so long as the overdose is maintained. With lower doses, these side effects disappear. Each person should work with her doctor to find the ideal level of hormone that is best for her.

PHYSICAL CHANGES IN MEN

As we've said, impotence is *not* a normal part of aging. "Impotence" can mean anything from being incapable of erection some of the time to a total incapacity for erection. Just as it is with women, a man's lack of ability for arousal can be related to stress, depression, disease, or medication. If impotence occurs, it's important to find out *why* it's occurring and then to treat the condition. Among men, and sometimes among their doctors, however, there seems to be a great deal of misunderstanding about impotence. As we've said before, a universal feature of growing older is a gradual slowing down of the sexual response. Some men tend to interpret this slowing down as a sign of oncoming sexual problems or impotence—which it is not.

Most older men enjoy an active sexual life. One of the original authors of the *Kinsey Report* on male sexuality, Dr. Clyde E. Martin, found current evidence to support the theory that men remain sexually vigorous well into their later years. In 1981, at the National Institute on Aging's Gerontology Research Center, Dr. Martin found that a group of the "most active," normal, healthy men age sixty and over had intercourse an average of once every 3.9 days. The "least active" group had sexual intercourse no more frequently than once every 60.8 days.

Older men usually require a longer time to achieve full erection—an equivalent to the older woman's taking longer to lubricate—four minutes, for instance, instead of thirty seconds. Masters and Johnson have established that normally healthy men do *not* lose their ability to achieve and maintain an erection as a result of aging. When a man loses that ability, it's almost always because of psychological reasons, nonsexual physical problems, or an illness.

A complete absence of erections in older men strongly indicates an organic problem, says Dr. Eric Pfeiffer, a professor of psychiatry at the University of Southern Florida Medical Center and director of the Suncoast Gerontology Center. It's possible that diabetes, severe arteriosclerosis in the pelvic vessels, or extensive pelvic surgery has caused men not to be able to have an erection. Dr. Pfeiffer suggests that in such instances, patients and their doctors should consider newer surgical techniques that utilize an inflatable implanted penile prosthesis.

A Change in Ejaculation

After a man's experience with ejaculation has been consistent for many years, it's unsettling when the quality and quantity of ejaculation changes, which it does for most men sixty-five or older. Eventually in an older man, orgasm occurs in one stage rather than two (many older men report that they no longer have the sensation of "orgasmic inevitability" that immediately precedes climax), and the amount of seminal fluid is smaller and comes out with less force. Also, the time it takes after ejaculation for the man to have another erection and climax increases with age.

The biggest problems that are caused by these physiological changes are psychological. "Men scare themselves," says Myrna Lewis. "They're particularly concerned with their masculinity and can easily get depressed at the prospect that they're no longer the men they were."

Tragically, some of these men withdraw from sexual activity at a time when their wives have not lost the ability or the desire for sex. Instead of adapting to the pleasurable sex they could be having, these men compensate by dropping their libido rather than exploring the possibilities for pleasure with their mate. Unfortunately, if they consult their doctors, some of them will be told that they should "expect" to lose interest in sex "at their age." As a result, undiagnosed disease states are often overlooked, or normal responses that could be compensated for are never understood.

Masters and Johnson have pointed out that almost all problems with impotence are psychological, not physical. They've made a practical suggestion that older men should remember that it's not necessary to ejaculate every time they have intercourse. If they hold back instead of feeling forced to ejaculate, they can have more frequent sex and feel more in command of their behavior. If reduced ejaculation doesn't worry either the man or the woman, it won't interfere with their pleasure. If anything, sometimes the man's ability to maintain an erection without ejaculation may add to his own and his partner's sexual pleasure.

Special Male Problems

A purely physical problem with erection and ejaculation may occur when a man has a diagnosed and controlled case of diabetes. The onset of diabetes is common in old age, and although the disease itself doesn't lower sexual drive, it can cause impotence. Although the impotence is sometimes permanent, more often than not it can be reversed and controlled by proper diet or medication. (Women with diabetes, by the way, don't seem to have the same sexual problems that men do. Studies have shown that women with advanced diabetes are as normal sexually as women without it.)

Prostate problems can also cause problems with impotence, but doctors say that this is the exception, not the rule. Men with prostate problems often have to have surgery on the enlarged gland at the base of the urethra. This gland produces the fluid that helps to nourish and transport sperm as it's ejaculated. Without prostatic fluid, a man can still enjoy sex, but he is infertile. Because the prostrate gland surrounds the urethra, it can press on the urethra and block the flow of the urine when it enlarges. If this condition isn't treated, it can cause a backup of the urine and lead to kidney and bladder infections. The enlargement of the gland can also cause pain during erection and ejaculation.

Three different techniques are commonly used in a prostatectomy. They are:

- The suprapubic operation, where the gland is removed through an abdominal incision.
- The transurethral resection (TUR), where the doctor performs the operation by threading an instrument through the penis. This is the most common surgical technique. It leaves no scar because there's no incision.
- The perineal, where the surgeon makes an incision between the anus and the scrotum. This technique is more likely to cause physical impotence than the other two techniques.

Doctors say that aside from radical prostatectomies (not transurethral), which commonly lead to sexual dysfunction, impotence from prostate surgery is the exception, not the rule. They say that sometimes the impotence is psychological, not physiological, following surgery.

Currently researchers are experimenting with a laser that would be used in a doctor's office to destroy the excess tissue in the prostate gland without requiring any incision.

Keeping the Sperm in the Body
After a prostatectomy, about half the men who have had this surgery ejaculate their semen back into the bladder instead of out through the penis. This reverse ejaculation is harmless, and the semen is reabsorbed by the body. Nevertheless, if a man hasn't fully discussed and understood exactly what is happening to him physiologically, he can be worried and adversely affected by the physiological changes. Also, unless he talks with his doctor about the way he will function sexually after the

surgery, he may assume that he'll no longer be as potent as he used to be. Sometimes patients avoid the operation or medication following the operation because they're not informed about the risks and benefits involved.

Fear of Sexual Failure

"Abby" had been noticing that her father, "Jake Goldman," a trim seventy-eight-year-old, was getting fat around his waist and abdomen. After having been a widower for seven years, Jake had been remarried for nearly two years, so Abby thought he must be enjoying his new wife's cooking. "I should have wondered more about it than I did," says Abby, "because he'd always been very trim—and his weight had never varied in all the years I'd known him.

"I also noticed that he was constantly in the bathroom when he and Emma were visiting me. If Emma hadn't been with him, I might have said something or asked about it, but since she was there, I figured they were talking about it.

"About three weeks or so after their last visit, Ben and I were on vacation when my son called to let us know that Grandpa had just gone into the hospital. Apparently he had been having prostate problems—and he'd let it go until it was almost too late. As a result, he almost died!

"Fortunately, he went to see my friend Steve, who is a urologist, and Steve had him admitted to the hospital on an emergency basis. He'd been walking around with a bladder that was so full he'd gotten uremic poisoning. Steve said he'd never seen such serious uremic poisoning, and that he'd never had to drain such an enormous quantity of it. He couldn't believe what my father had been walking around with!

"My father is a very bright, highly educated man, but, because of bad experiences over the years, he's very stubborn when it comes to doctors. He thought just about anything was better than going to a doctor.

"They did prostatic surgery on him twice, and for a while there, he had to catheterize himself once a day. Apparently it's much better now, but he's continued to turn down medicine that Steve wanted to give him.

"We were talking about it the last time he visited. I was urging him to take the medicine, but he said, 'You know there are side effects to that stuff! It makes you impotent!'

"I was really surprised. It hadn't occurred to me that at the age of seventy-eight he'd be concerned about impotence to the point that he would refuse medicine that might make his condition better."

Looking for Reasons

If a man who's otherwise healthy and free of extra stress becomes unable to sustain an erection even if he gets one, he should suspect his medications. Certainly his antihypertensives, tranquilizers, or antidepressants could be responsible. Anyone having problems on these medications should consult a doctor. Usually, if these drugs are changed or discontinued, a man's potency will return. He should *not* discontinue the medications without his doctor's knowledge, however, since the absence of certain medications can be life-threatening.

Another factor in male impotence, besides medications, may well be the use of alcohol. Alcohol is known to damage sexual capacity and to make a man incapable of achieving or maintaining an erection.

ATTITUDES ABOUT YOURSELF

Men and women alike learn to cope with certain emotional reactions to the way they look and feel and perform as they age. As it is with every other stage of life, there are new adjustments and new questions.

Just as people do when they're younger, older people also worry about their attractiveness and desirability. Since age has not been greatly lauded in our culture, being seventy or eighty doesn't sound appealing to a lot of people who have reached that age. As you might expect from earlier patterns, says Myrna Lewis, older men worry about their sexual performance. They don't worry about changes in their faces or bodies. They can accept their pot bellies if they feel they're still able to perform sexually. Women, on the other hand, become very concerned about appearance—about the way their skin looks or their bottoms sag. Whether a woman can or can't perform sexually doesn't worry her; she's concerned about how she looks and often has difficulty adjusting to the changes in her appearance.

"This mirrors the way in which we quite automatically slot people in early life," says Ms. Lewis. "Men are rewarded for their performance, and women are rewarded for their appearance. Women who successfully make that transition from fifty to seventy, however, risk becoming idolized. They become grand dames. They reach a level of security because they accept themselves so fully, and they don't have to give a damn what anyone thinks!"

Sexual Fantasies and Sexual Pleasure
Sometimes, when older persons lose partners, or when their partners become inactive for a variety of reasons, they lose their own zest for life. Sometimes they feel that it is "dirty" or inappropriate for them to masturbate or satisfy themselves sexually. But, in fact, doctors point out the benefits of maintaining sexual vitality. Besides being relaxing, sexual activity and orgasm relieve tension, get the blood flowing, and keep you in contact with your own vital spirit. Sometimes actively using your sexual fantasies for fun and pleasure provides a healthy release and a satisfying experience.

Geriatric Community Health Consultant Virginia

Barrett interviewed people sixty-five and older about their sexual fantasies. Everyone she interviewed had sexual fantasies—and many of her respondents activated their fantasies into various levels of reality. One widower, a retired executive whom she interviewed, was in his late seventies and lived on Long Island. "He and his wife had had a very active sex life," Ms. Barrett said in an interview. "He missed her, but he wasn't interested in getting into a new relationship. Still, he needed an outlet for his sexual energy. He'd been a prominent businessman and was still good friends with his former partner. The two of them would go to Forty-second Street in New York City at ten o'clock in the morning to see pornographic films, and then go out to lunch.

"Weren't you scared of being mugged in Times Square?" Ms. Barrett asked her respondent.

"First of all, drug addicts aren't up at nine-thirty in the morning, and besides, eighty percent of the other people in the theater were retired people," he said. "They're not down-and-outers. They're people like me."

The dapper executive told Ms. Barrett that after seeing a sexually explicit film, he'd spend the next few nights thinking about those scenes. It made him feel good, and he believed it kept him healthy.

Ms. Barrett also talked with women in their eighties and nineties who had active sexual fantasies. One woman in her mid-eighties, who volunteered at the local library, enjoyed watching the young men in the library and had fantasies about them following her home. She also enjoyed reading semipornographic books whenever they came across her path.

Ms. Barrett said that many women and men over sixty-five with whom she talked either felt too guilty to masturbate or felt that they needed an excuse if they did. "They grew up in an era when that was a no-no," she says. "A lot of women without partners would like

sexual activity in their lives, but they feel too guilty
about it. They do want to talk about it, however, and
they want advice. They need to hear that it's a healthy
thing.''

SEX AND THE DISEASES OF OLD AGE

Heart Disease
Many older people with cardiac problems or high blood
pressure are afraid that if they have sexual intercourse,
they'll have a heart attack (or another heart attack). The
assumption is so strong with many people that they don't
ask their doctor about it. If the doctor isn't aware of the
patient's concern, or has stereotypes himself about sexual behavior in older people, the subject might never
be discussed. In fact, except for very severe cases, doctors say, normal sexual activity can be beneficial for the
heart. The slightly increased heart rate, blood pressure,
and oxygen consumption can be excellent for the system. Also, lovemaking reduces stress and encourages
relaxation, which are also good for the heart.

In her book *The Best Years of Your Life*, Dr. Miriam
Stoppard suggests that since people who have had heart
attacks have to be careful not to get overtired, it might
be better to have sexual relations in the morning after
a good night's rest instead of in the evening. She also
suggests that lying side by side, face to face, is less
strenuous than the ''missionary position''—and that
finding other positions can also help avoid muscle
cramps and tension.

Arthritis
Dr. Stoppard suggests that patterns of lovemaking can
also be changed to accommodate yourself to discomforts caused by arthritis. ''Painful, stiff joints may make
the ordinary face-to-face position difficult, but the
adoption of a new position—such as with the woman

on top (if the male is arthritic)—can often bring success," she says. "Taking painkilling drugs before having sex can also help. Even if the problems involved in making love are so severe that you decide to forgo full intercourse, you should never abstain from indulging in other sexual activities if you and/or your partner desire them. Physical closeness through touching and caresses can provide a great deal of comfort and reassurance."

USE IT OR LOSE IT—THEN USE IT AGAIN!

Another big problem for older people sometimes occurs when they have stopped their sexual activity for a number of years. Just as your muscles stay in shape when you maintain an active schedule of exercise, so does your reproductive system stay in shape when it's used. Often when it's not used, your penis or vagina can have what's called atrophy of disuse. The longer an older person has abstained from sexual activity, the less likely he or she is to have such activity restored on a regular basis.

Don't be discouraged, however, if you have been abstinent for some time and wish to be active again someday. Dr. Panter tells of just such a person, "Mrs. Jamison," who came in to see him for a Pap smear six months after her husband's death. She was a handsome woman in her sixties at the time, had had a normal sex life with her husband, and was in good shape gynecologically. When she came in again six months later, Dr. Panter asked her about her sex life. She answered that she wasn't having sex. "I'm from the old school," she told him. "I've dated a few people, but I haven't wanted to sleep with anyone."

Dr. Panter told her that he noticed that her vagina was beginning to become narrow because she wasn't using it. "It's like if you kept your arm in a sling," Dr. Panter said. "Your muscles would get thin and weak."

Dr. Panter suggested that she go on estrogen to stop the atrophy, but she said she didn't want to. Four years later, with no estrogen and no sex, the woman's vagina had narrowed significantly. During the examination, Dr. Panter had to use a small size speculum—the kind appropriate for young girls fifteen and sixteen. Six months later, however, when the same woman came in for another checkup, she said, "You've got to change my name on your records!" When Dr. Panter asked why, she said, "Three months ago, I met a forty-six-year-old man, and he fell in love with me!" Thinking of the twenty-two-year age difference, Dr. Panter asked why she married him instead of just living with him. "Well," she responded, "I pointed out to him that I was old enough to be his mother, but he said he loved me and wanted to marry me. He signed a prenuptial agreement, and he treats me with respect and trust."

When Dr. Panter asked about their sexual relationship, she smiled and said, "Everything is all right now, but the first few times we had intercourse it was very painful. After about two weeks, it began to feel all right again."

"That's an example of atrophy that can be corrected by using an organ again," said Dr. Panter. "It was like an atrophied muscle that had been exercised again. It was accomplished with no hormones. She feels as comfortable sexually now as she ever did, and she doesn't need hormones for her sexuality."

ASK YOUR DOCTOR

Remember, if you run into trouble sexually, most likely it's because of circumstances in your life, such as depression, disease, or medication. Don't assume that sexual difficulties are a normal thing. If you want to have a satisfying sexual relationship, there's no reason you shouldn't have one, no matter your age.

If sexuality is important to you, don't wait for your doctor to ask you about your sexual functioning. "Most doctors won't ask, so raise it yourself," advises Myrna Lewis. "They've not had any courses on human sexuality in medical schools until recently—and practically no medical school will teach them the sexual side effects of any medication or information about the polypharmacy of geriatrics. Older people have to lead their physicians into the twentieth century in terms of the pharmacy of geriatrics!"

As Myrna Lewis points out, if you raise the subject of sexuality, then at least you'll get your doctor thinking about it. If Aldomet (methyldopa) is indicated because of high blood pressure, for instance, he'll know, if you've mentioned sex, that Aldomet causes sexual problems—and that it matters to you.

If your doctor prescribes antihypertensives, tranquilizers, or antidepressants for you, ask him how these medications will affect your sexual functioning.

When your doctor gives you a new prescription, ask, "How is this going to affect my sex life? What are the sexual side effects of this drug?" If you ask such questions, they alert the doctor to consider the sexual side effects of your treatment. If he doesn't know about the sexual side effects of the medication, ask him to look it up in a drug reference.

If the medications are going to have a negative effect on your sex life, then ask your doctor what alternative medications would be effective. What are your risks and what are your benefits? Get answers to your questions and work things out with your doctor and your partner. There may be some situations where you have no alternative, but those are few and far between.

In the meantime, you can draw hope from Dr. Alexander Leaf, who studied the physical effects of aging and visited the three places in the world where human beings are said to live the longest. After going back to Harvard Medical School from his travels to the Hunza region of Pakistan, a village in Ecuador, and the Soviet republic of Georgia in the Caucasus Mountains, Dr. Leaf wrote in his book *Youth in Old Age*, ''Sexual activity is, of course, not a requirement for long life. But since sex is one of the gifts nature has provided to add enjoyment, zest, and fulfillment to our existence, it plays a significant role in our lives. Since my thesis is that the well-adjusted, happy, confident, and socially productive person is one likely to live long, in this context, a continuing and healthy sexual adjustment is important through the total life span.''

YOUR MEDICATIONS AND SEXUAL ACTIVITY*

Because these medications address your circulatory system or your nervous system, they also may affect some aspects of your sexuality. As with any drug effect, the nature and degree to which sexual experience is affected will vary a great deal from one individual to the next. If you are experiencing any sexual difficulties, it may be related to a medication you are taking. Make sure to consult your doctor if you suspect such a possibility.

DRUG   POSSIBLE SIDE EFFECTS

	REDUCED LIBIDO	REDUCED POTENCY	IMPAIRED EJACULATION	PROLONGED, PAINFUL ERECTIONS	DELAYED ORGASM IN WOMEN
acetazolamide	✔	✔			
alcohol		✔			✔
amphetamine	✔	✔			
anti-depressants	✔	✔	✔		
anti-histamines	✔	✔			

	REDUCED LIBIDO	REDUCED POTENCY	IMPAIRED EJACULATION	PROLONGED, PAINFUL ERECTIONS	DELAYED ORGASM IN WOMEN
atropinelike drugs (anticholinergics)		✓	✓		
beta-blockers	✓	✓			
cimetidine	✓	✓			
clofibrate	✓	✓			
clonidine	✓	✓	✓		
dextroamphetamine	✓	✓			
diazepam	✓		✓		
diethylstilbestrol	✓	✓			
digitalis preparations		✓			
disopyramide		✓			
disulfiram		✓			
estrogens	✓ (in men)				
fenfluramine	✓	✓			
haloperidol		✓		✓	
methyldopa	(impotence)				
Diuretics:					
ethacrynic acid		✓			
furosemide		✓			
Antihypertensives:					
guanethidine	(for women) ✓	✓	✓	✓	
reserpine	(for women) ✓		✓		

*Adapted from *The Essential Guide to Prescription Drugs* by James W. Long, M.D., 4th Ed., Harper & Row, New York, 1985.

CHAPTER 11

Extending Your Life—Folk Remedies,
Quack Cures, Nutrition, and Exercise

"Experts tend to under-predict and laypersons to fantasize about the future.

"I sometimes think it might be equally helpful, as the twentieth century gallops ahead, to proceed by outright divination. In whimsical deference thereto I have cast the *I Ching*, that ancient Chinese system of divination in which yarrow stalks are cast and the meaning of the pattern of their fall in relation to the question posed is read from the ancient text, the Book of Changes, which is the *I Ching*. As recently as the seventeenth century great Lord Yamaga built the Japanese samurai into the finest fighting force in Asia by teaching them strategy that accorded with a special interpretation of the *I Ching*. So let's take a look. In response to my question, 'Will significant life span extension be achieved in the next five to fifteen years?,' the yarrow stalks have fallen into the following favorable hexagram,

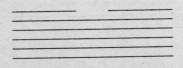

called the Kuai hexagram, whereof the *I Ching* text says, "This hexagram signifies on one hand a breakthrough after a long accumulation of tension, as a swollen river breaks through its dikes, or in the manner of a cloudburst."

The *I Ching* seems to describe what we have come to recognize as a paradigm change, either scientific or social or both. With such an auspicious readout added to what we already know about the biology of aging, optimism is in order."

—ROY L. WOLFORD, M.D., in *Maximum Life Span*

At the age of eighty-five, retired teacher Rose Anderson has experienced a series of strokes, heart attacks, and problems with her vision due to cataracts. Among her operations, Rose had surgery on both carotid arteries. What might keep others down for months, however, seems barely to deter her. Usually within several days to two weeks after an operation, she's seen tooling around her Stanwood, Washington, retirement community on her electrified Diablo scooter, stopping to visit with neighbors and friends, who jump out of the way when they see her speeding toward them with what they think is reckless abandon (and what she thinks is perfect control). When Rose passes out in church, which happens frequently these days because of her blood pressure, she's furious if she wakes up in the hospital. "Just leave me alone for a few minutes and I'll be fine!" she's instructed her husband, sister, and friends. "Don't call the ambulance! Everybody worries too much!"

After her last cataract operation, Rose, who is one to look on the bright side, said enthusiastically, "I can read for two whole minutes without my vision blurring!"

Recently, one day after church, when she *hadn't* passed out, she was talking with a woman who had just turned one hundred.

"I've never been sick a day in my life!" the woman said proudly, "and I've never been in the hospital!"

"That's wonderful!" Rose said. "What a blessing!"

"It's because I've always done what God told me to do!" the woman volunteered. "I've always done what's right."

"Well, I've always done what God told me to do, too," Rose responded, "and I've always done what's right. Why do you think I've had everything under the sun go wrong with me?"

The centurian thought for a moment and then looked carefully at Rose's pink-toned skin, white hair, and large brown eyes. "Do you eat the skin on chicken?" she asked.

"Yes," Rose answered.

"Well, you shouldn't eat the skin on chicken."

Everyone has a theory. While one says it's chicken without the skin and another that it's yogurt and a glass of wine daily, others maintain that the only difference between whether we live to be 73 or 105 are the genes with which we were born.

Currently, the outside possibility for any human life is about 115 years. That's the "maximum" life span— and very few of us get that far. Those who get anywhere close are thoroughly queried. If a 105-year-old says she drinks a glass of brandy every evening, we decide that maybe we should try a brandy a night. When the Azer-baijans of the Georgian Republic of Russia, who were said to live to 130, reported that they ate fresh fruits, vegetables, and corn meal, drank two glasses of butter-milk a day and a small quantity of red wine with low alcohol content, word went around that this was the diet to follow. When a prolific writer says that sex or relax-ation or a daily walk is what works, many of us listen with attention. Certainly, myths about how to stave off aging, how to keep vigorous and extend our lives, are of keen interest to all of us. The search for that illusive fountain of youth is one that holds allure for nearly everyone.

ANTIAGING GIMMICKS THAT DON'T WORK

Our desire to feel better, live longer, to be more vital, and to look younger sometimes makes us cling desperately to easy answers. According to a report issued in May 1984 by the Subcommittee on Health and Long-Term Care of the House Select Committee on Aging, "antiaging" products alone bring in about $2 billion a year and are the fastest-growing segment of today's medical quackery.

The promotion and sales of useless remedies that promise relief from aging and from chronic and critical health conditions exceed $10 billion a year, according to the report that documented the results of a four-year investigation. This "quackery" has as a common denominator, it said, "the element of conscious deceit and the absence of, and in most cases the total disregard for, scientific proof." What's more, this business of providing medical remedies known to be false, for profit, is growing at an alarming rate—probably more than 12 percent a year.

The committee found that older people were particularly vulnerable to health frauds perpetrated through the mail; testimony indicated that more than 60 percent of those victimized by mail scams were elderly.

During the course of its investigation, the committee reviewed hundreds of products that promised to arrest or reverse aging and alleviate conditions commonly associated with growing older. One product, "Young Again," advertised by a Connecticut firm, promised to "make you look ten to fifteen years younger in just sixty seconds" by causing "wrinkles, lines, and crow's-feet [to] disappear." After an analysis of "Young Again," Dr. Roger B. Hickler, director of the Division of Geriatric Medicine at the University of Massachusetts and assistant professor of Dermatology at Harvard Medical School, said that the product contained essentially the same ingredients found at a beach—sand, water, and some oxides thrown in. He said the lotion "failed to smooth away lines and wrinkles," and that some of the substances were skin irritants known to cause allergic reactions in susceptible individuals.

A company called Nature Life Products advertised a "No Aging Plan" in 1981, and claimed that its product, "RNA + 13," would improve memory and alertness, increase energy, improve heart function, reduce breathlessness and fatigue, increase resistance to viral diseases, smooth out wrinkles, combat skin disorders, and make some people appear ten to fifteen years younger. It also stated that in some cases "RNA + 13" would actually reverse tissue degeneration. The advertisement said that "many startling discoveries about RNA's effects on aging and disease have been reported in respected scientific journals." Dr. Sorell L. Schwartz, professor of Pharmacology at Georgetown University School of Medicine, who reviewed the product, which is a multivitamin preparation containing iron and ribonucleic acid (RNA), said that the claims for "RNA + 13" "are massive and more outrageously false and misleading than any I have seen for similar products."

Many products the committee investigated claimed to increase energy, restore hair, and/or rejuvenate skin. One hair-restorative that contained vitamins, minerals, and a substance called para-aminobenzoic acid was considered not only ineffective but dangerous by Dr. Alvin Segelman, chairman of the Department of Pharmacognosy at Rutgers University, who said that not only will "para-aminobenzoic acid aid in the growth of bacterial infections, but it will also *reverse the beneficial effects of antibacterial sulfa drugs*, which are often administered to people suffering from bacterial infections in order to clear up these infections." A pep pill called "Lift" was found to contain enormous amounts of caffeine, yet this information did not appear on the label of the product. Dr. Segelman pointed out that if a user of "Lift" took four tablets before each meal, as recommended, he would be consuming the equivalent of three to five cups of strong coffee three times a day. He concluded that the use of this product by people who should not be consuming caffeine (heart patients, for example) could lead to serious medical and health problems. He also said that at $8.95 a bottle, about one week's supply, "It seems to me that this is a very expensive way for the consumer to pay for what is essentially equivalent to cups of coffee."

The investigation by the committee also found that older people are enticed by hundreds of magic cures and dangerous diets that claim to cure cancer and arthritis. They estimated that elderly people spent $4 to $5 billion on fraudulent cancer cures and $2 billion a year on arthritis remedies. The reliance of cancer patients on unproven remedies, according to the report, is generated by a variety of factors, including the fact that there is only limited knowledge of the nature of cancer and the progress that has been made in cancer therapy. Cancer is a dreaded disease, and when diagnosed, it inspires desperation. Similarly, people with arthritis are vulnerable to quackery, according to the Arthritis Foundation, because presently there's no cure for it, and because there is tremendous pain associated with the disease. In addition, symptoms of arthritis come and go, allowing people to connect a disappearance with a phony remedy they have just been taking. Some of the examples reviewed by the committee included a "miracle spike" to cure cancer and diabetes that sold for $300. The people who bought it weren't getting any reliable help; what they were getting was a penny's worth of barium chloride to wear on a chain around their necks. Other fantastic devices that were sold to older people included the "Congo Kit," two hemp mittens that when worn were supposed to cure arthritis; an "inducto-scope" supposed to cure arthritis through magnetic induction; and a bag of "moon dust," also an arthritis cure, which was just a bag of plain sand.

Even when the products are innocuous, they encourage victims of serious diseases to treat themselves with ineffective products and to waste time and money by delaying effective medical care. Often, when good medical treatment could have been effective early in the progression of the disease, by the time it's sought, it's too late.

"Over 75 percent of the products reviewed by the committee were found to be dangerous or potentially harmful," says Representative Claude Pepper, chairman of the Subcommittee on Health and Long-Term Care. "In addition to the loss of money paid for nonexistent cures, individuals who purchase these products are exposing themselves to hazards ranging from blindness to the acceleration of cancer, aggravation of arthritis, convulsions, heart palpitations, insulin shock, and death."

People who testified at the congressional hearings often explained how desperate they felt when they allowed themselves to be led into false promises. "I know that I was foolish," said one sixty-one-year-old witness who paid more than $2,000 to a health-food "doctor" (with a Ph.D. in engineering) to cure her husband's cancer. The "doctor" advised that she keep her husband away from hospitals and hospital food (because they were "poison") and give him a diet of wheat grass juice, watermelon rind juice, and the juice of green vegetables. "I know it now. But my husband and I were married for thirty-seven years, and when he got sick, I was looking for magic. Their false promise of hope may have actually shortened my husband's few numbered days on this earth."

When the consequences aren't so dire, older people who've been victimized simply feel embarrassed at how gullible they can be.

"Janet Edwards" told me that a number of years ago

she paid $1,200 over six months' time to a "physical therapist" who claimed to teach people how to keep their bodies firm and youthful-looking well into their nineties. "The main ingredient of her "program" called for tightening your buttocks when you were standing, walking, or driving," eighty-year-old Janet said recently. "Sometimes, still, when I'm at a red light, I'll automatically tighten my buttocks like she told me to do. When I do it, I realize what I've done and feel like a fool all over again.

"She might just as well have told me to throw salt over my shoulder and hang garlic outside my front door so I could live to be one hundred. It was ridiculous. I was really hoodwinked."

The report by the Committee on Aging was careful to say that they had no intention of disparaging every unproven remedy—recognizing that "the practice of healing continues to evolve" and that "some of what is unproven may yet prove of benefit." There are people, however, who carelessly call alternative avenues of therapy "quackery" because they don't fit into current accepted medical practices—or because evidence of their effectiveness is incomplete. Many years ago, for instance, some of the doctors who experimented with certain low-salt or low-cholesterol diets to control disease were called "quacks" by colleagues who pointed to contradictions or lack of evidence of benefits. When experiments began in biofeedback and other relaxation techniques, they looked "crazy" to many medical professionals. Today it's recognized that many of those so-called quacks were on the right track. The medical profession now openly acknowledges the importance of diet and stress reduction in reducing heart disease and the effectiveness of biofeedback in treating many stress-related disorders, most notably headaches, hypertension, irritable bowel disease, and immune system deficiencies.

In the same way, some of today's "alternative" approaches may have real benefits and may one day be recognized as perfectly valid by the medical community. What's important is that all avenues of communication remain open. If, for instance, you have cancer and you want to go on a macrobiotic diet because you believe it will be good for you, let your medical doctor know exactly what you're doing and why so that he can discuss risks and benefits with you and give you appropriate support and care. You may decide to combine a traditional medical therapy with hypnosis, diet, massage, and acupuncture. You may learn biofeedback techniques or practice meditation at the same time you're receiving chemotherapy. Keep an open mind as to what works and what doesn't. Look at the track record—which should be more than a small pamphlet or a few testimonials in an advertisement. If you want to try something that hasn't been proven, don't fool yourself into believing it's a certainty. Acknowledge its experimental nature. You have every right to be a pioneer if you want to be. You also have the right to try several different approaches simultaneously. Just make sure you understand what your options are and what the risks are. Take time to research and comprehend what you're doing, but don't be afraid to take action on your own behalf. Ask questions and expect answers.

Certainly, you are free to act in your own best interests. But don't be persuaded that you will be "cured" by anything called Moon Dust or Blue Fire—or that you will live to be 102 if you wear an amulet around your neck. So far, nothing is "proven" or "foolproof" when it comes to ensuring long life. Your body is a complex system—one to be respected. If you plan to use an "alternative" medicine, vitamins, or other food supplements, again be sure to tell your medical doctor what you are doing. He or she may not approve, but at least you won't get into problems with multiple medications if your medical counselors are aware of your program.

Unfortunately, it is not difficult to counteract your medical treatment, or worse, to injure yourself with the unwise use of self-treatment.

APPROACHES TO HEALTH AND LONG LIFE THAT DO WORK

While there's a great deal we don't know, and while it's clear that there are no easy answers, the possibility of extending the life span may become a reality sooner than we could imagine. Even if we don't see the life span stretch to 150, 180, or even 200 years, our prospects for living to a healthy and productive old age are far better today than they were in the past.

Researchers who have studied the aging process tell us that good diet, exercise, life-style, personal relationships, and social factors in our lives have been underestimated in terms of the important role they play. And while certain ninety-year-olds who smoke cigars and sip cocktails every evening defy the rules, it does appear that lowered stress levels, avoidance of tobacco, having some control over our environment, adapting well to change, and feeling loved all play an important part in helping us live longer.

In a review of literature on aging, Dr. John Rowe and Robert Kahn, a research scientist at the Institute for Social Research, say that they believe the role of physiological aging has been exaggerated when it comes to age-associated losses. On the other hand, they say, the modifying effects of life-style, habits, diet, and an array of psychosocial factors have been either ignored or attributed to differences in genetic endowment.

"Factors of diet and exercise, nutrition, and life-style seem to have been underestimated or ignored as potential moderators of the aging process," says Dr. Rowe. "If so, the prospects for reversing functional losses with age are vastly improved, and the risk of adverse health outcomes is reduced.''

THE ROLE OF NUTRITION

Many of the declines that we have associated with aging may, in fact, be directly related to poor nutrition. According to Dr. Jeffrey Blumberg, assistant director of the USDA Human Nutrition Center on Aging at Tufts University, poor nutrition appears to strongly influence the functional decline in a wide variety of the body's organ systems. Nutrition may also be an important influence on progressive changes in body composition associated with aging, such as the loss of lean body mass and bone, and it may be directly related to the physiological decline in the immune system. This decline has commonly been blamed on aging. Evidence also demonstrates that nutrition is linked to many chronic diseases afflicting older people in this country.

Unfortunately, malnourishment is all too common among the elderly. According to Dr. Blumberg, national and regional surveys over the past ten years have found that some 40 percent of older Americans are malnourished. Some of these people are malnourished because of hunger and a lack of food, while others have ill-chosen diets that may contain enough food but not enough of the right calories or micronutrients people need to stay healthy.

Federally subsidized programs such as Meals on Wheels and hot-lunch programs at senior-citizen centers are beginning to address the issues of hunger and malnutrition for many older people. Health-care workers are also beginning to focus on diet and nutrition as a vital component of the health-care delivery system for older people. But even more attention needs to be paid to this problem.

While many low-income people have a difficult time eating well, middle-class or affluent people suffer malnourishment, too. Sometimes a multitude of non-nutritional factors, including physical activity and medications, can influence food intakes and the ways the body utilizes nutrients. Inadequate nutrition can result from the loss of taste, the side effects of drugs, or from disease. And when older people are lonely and depressed, malnourishment may not be a matter of energy or economics. In his Pulitzer Prize–winning book, *Why Survive? Being Old in America*, Dr. Robert Butler tells of a ninety-five-year-old retired corporation executive who lived in an exclusive apartment complex. "He had outlived friends and relatives," Dr. Butler writes. "He had an income over $900 a month, and $300,000 in assets, yet he was starving to death. His memory had become hazy and he forgot his mealtimes. No one realized he was subsisting on a few sweets and tea."

"When we talk about inadequate calories or micronutrients," says Dr. Blumberg, "we're talking about the same kind of problem among affluent whites as among impoverished and isolated people from other ethnic groups. The problems come from diets that are not balanced or not wisely enough selected."

While malnutrition is a problem for older people, so is obesity. As Shakespeare said in *The Merchant of Venice*, "They are as sick that surfeit with too much as they that starve with nothing." Older people who continue to struggle with weight control should be very careful about how they diet. Diets that are extreme, such as all-protein diets, can be very harmful, as can fasting. Often, problems of being overweight are due to eating the wrong foods—too much fat, too much sugar, too much salt. If you are overweight, you would probably do well to look at the dietary guidelines recommended by the American Heart Association. They recommend a reduced saturated fat, salt, and cholesterol intake—a suggestion good for people of any weight. They also recommend that you consume a wide variety of foods, with your protein intake being approximately fifteen percent of your calories, and carbohydrates, fifty to fifty-five percent. The American Cancer Association recommends that you also cut down on your total fat intake and eat more high-fiber foods, such as fruits, vegetables, and whole-grains cereals. They say that your diet should include foods rich in vitamins A and C and vegetables such as cabbage, broccoli, brussels sprouts, kohlrabi, and cauliflower. They advise moderation in consuming salt-cured, smoked, and nitrite-cured foods, such as hot dogs, and, like the American Heart Association, recommend moderate consumption of alcoholic beverages.

A Well-Balanced Diet

If you wonder whether you're eating well and giving your body the nourishment it needs, think about the basics of good nutrition. It's easy, in day-to-day living, to lose track of them.

Ask yourself, "Do I eat a variety of nutritious foods? Do I eat in moderation?" A good diet will include plenty of fiber, which you can get in fruits, vegetables, cereals, whole grains, and enriched bread. In the course of a week, you should also try to eat fish, poultry, small amounts of meat, an egg, dried peas and beans, and low-fat milk. As Jane Brody points out in *Jane Brody's Nutrition Book*, potatoes and legumes (peanuts or peanut butter, soybeans, kidney, navy, pinto and lima beans, seeds, and dried peas) are wonderful sources of nutrition. If you don't care for meat, you can get the complete protein you need in combining legumes with oats, sesame seeds, wheat, brown rice, corn, and barley. These products are not expensive, and they're good for your health.

It's also extremely important that you drink water. Water is particularly necessary as you age. According to Drs. Cary S. Kart and Seamus P. Metress, authors of *Nutrition, the Aged and Society*, dehydration is common in older people. Sometimes it's the result of disease, and sometimes it's simply the result of minimal water intake. "All metabolic reactions require water," they write, "even small changes. You need water for swallowing, for digesting your food, and eliminating it. Water also functions to regulate your body temperature through sweating and reducing the load on your kidneys. It's not uncommon for symptoms of water imbalance to be accepted as characteristic of old age. They're not. Water imbalance may be characterized by apathy, body weakness, depression, mental confusion, or difficulty in swallowing." If you drink enough water—which should be six to eight glasses a day—you can reverse these symptoms.

Don't try to substitute tea or coffee for water. They are *not* water, just because they're liquid. Tea and coffee are diuretics, so they can make you even more dehydrated than you already are. Drink water and drink fruit and vegetable juices that don't contain salt or sugar. Sometimes, in fact, if you're feeling tired or listless, a big glass of water can make you feel much better.

As you get older, most likely you'll eat smaller quantities of food because you'll have lower energy requirements. Lowering your food intake makes it all the more important for you to maintain quality in your diet by choosing the right, nutrient-dense foods. Studies have shown that many older individuals eat too few fruits and vegetables, especially those that are rich in vitamins A and C. And, according to Dr. Blumberg at Tufts University, despite the widespread use of enriched breads and cereals, low intakes of the B-complex vitamins are common among older individuals.

You can get the vitamins and minerals you need from the foods you eat. But if you decide to take vitamins, select supplements that are appropriate to your real needs. Keep in mind that vitamin bottles should list the percentage of the RDA on the label.

The following nutritional guides are based on the Recommended Dietary Allowances set by the National Academy of Science's National Research Council in 1980. These guidelines were set for people fifty-one years old and up, and as you know, a fifty-two-year-old and an eighty-nine-year-old simply will not have the same nutritional requirements. However, because there's a lack of adequate data about their needs, no official RDA has yet been set for people sixty-five and over.

Recommended Vitamins and Minerals
A (5,000 IU for men, 4,000 for women)—fish liver oils, eggs, butter, yellow vegetables, spinach, turnips, beet greens are good sources
B_1, thiamine (1.2 mg for men, 1 mg for women)—rice, bran, soy flour, mushrooms, turkey, nuts, liver
B_2, riboflavin (1.2 mg for men and women)—yeast, kidneys, avocados, wheat germ, bran
Niacin (16 mg for men, 13 mg for women)—yeast, chicken, peanuts, tuna, halibut, swordfish
B_6, pyridoxine (2 mg for men, 2 for women)—beef, pork, liver, brown rice, bananas, whole-grain cereal
Pantothenic acid (10 mg for men and women)—sources the same as B_6
Folic acid (400 mcg for men and women)—liver, dark green vegetables, dried beans, peanuts, wheat germ
B_{12}, cobalamin (3 mcg for men and women)—kidney, liver, milk, most cheese, fish, eggs
C, ascorbic acid (60 mg for men and women)—citrus fruit, strawberries, cranberries, broccoli, brussels sprouts, green pepper
D, calciferol (200 units for men and women)—direct sunlight, fortified milk, egg yolks, saltwater fish, liver
E, tocopherol (15 IU for men, 12 IU for women)—vegetable oils, nuts, legumes, whole-grain cereal

The National Academy of Sciences estimates that the following doses of minerals are a safe and adequate daily intake: Calcium, 800 milligrams for both men and women; phosphorus, 800 milligrams; magnesium, 350 milligrams for men, 300 for women. For the electrolytes, the NAS recommends a range: potassium, 1.8 to 5.6 grams; sodium, 1.1 to 3.3 grams; and chloride, 1.7 to 5.1 milligrams. Lesser amounts are needed of the trace minerals zinc, iron, iodine, copper, selenium, chromium, silicon, nickel, molybdenum, vanadium, cobalt, sulfur, manganese, and fluoride.

Researchers now involved in studies that eventually will lead to new RDA classifications for people sixty-five and older say that in general (unless you have a special diet, take medicines, or have a disease that would interfere) these recommended daily allowances are safe for you to take on a regular basis. They also say, however, that older people may need an increase in some specific nutrients and a decrease in others. The RDA for vitamin A and folate may be too high, for instance, since the absorption of A seems to increase with age and put older people at risk for vitamin A toxicity.* On the other hand, the RDA for vitamins B_6 and D and calcium may be too low because of age-related changes in the way they are metabolized. Some surveys report a third of the elderly consume only 0.5 milligrams of B_1 daily. A higher amount of B_1 and B_6 might be advised, and while the use of vitamin D supplements isn't generally recommended due to its potential for toxicity, it's been suggested that housebound or institutionalized people combine a low level of supplementation (400 I.U. daily) with increased exposure to sunlight whenever possible.

Although the NAS recommends 800 milligrams of calcium daily, a National Institutes of Health Consensus Conference in 1984 recommended a daily calcium in-

*The information regarding these nutrients comes from Dr. Jeffrey Blumberg, "Nutrient Requirements for the Healthy Elderly," *Contemporary Nutrition*, Vol. XI, No. 6, 1986.

take of 1000 milligrams in premenopausal and estrogen-treated postmenopausal women and 1500 milligrams in estrogen-deprived postmenopausal women.

Researchers also think that certain signs and symptoms associated with older age may be related to marginal zinc and chromium deficiencies, and that slightly higher intakes of zinc and chromium might be helpful.

Nutritional Deficiencies

A poor diet can be extremely detrimental. If the body gets out of balance, it attempts to correct that imbalance but often errs in some other direction as it does so. All too often, symptoms of these nutritional deficiencies are mistaken for new diseases and treated with medication, which further confuses the problem. In their book, *Nutrition, The Aged and Society*, Drs. Cary S. Kart and Seamus P. Metress discuss nutrient needs and relationships between nutrition and disease. Some of the ways they mention that an imbalance in your diet can cause health problems include the following:

- Deficiency of thiamine involves neurological manifestations and mood changes. Thiamine plays an important role in the process that changes glucose to energy. Poorly balanced or highly refined diets, stress, alcoholism, impaired intestinal absorption, or frequent use of diuretics are most often the factors that initiate thiamine deficiency.
- Riboflavin deficiency may be the most common deficiency among older people whose diets are low in meats and vegetables. This deficiency can cause visual impairment, sensitivity to bright light, and skin lesions.
- Mineral absorption can be made very inefficient by the use of laxatives and diarrhea that may result from that use. The lack of stomach acid due to antacid use

can reduce the stomach's capacity to dissolve minerals.

- The ratio of calcium to phosphorus in your diet is crucial in determining the balance of calcium in your body. If you have excessive amounts of phosphorus in your body, calcium is withdrawn from the bones to restore proper equilibrium. If, for instance, you regularly drink a lot of soda and eat a great deal of red meat, which are filled with phosphorus, or if you are on a long-term protein diet, the phosphorus levels in your body could get too high, and your body, trying to correct the imbalance, would draw calcium from your bones. Over time, this would result in a gradual reduction of bone density. Calcium deficiency leads to loss of muscle tone and decalcification of bones. You can add calcium to your diet by eating yogurt, sardines, canned salmon with bones, cooked spinach, broccoli, kale, or mustard greens, creamed cottage cheese, and oranges. Skim milk and whole milk are also good sources of calcium.

- Poor calcium intake may also be a significant factor in periodontal disease. There's some evidence that it can be reversed by adequate calcium intakes. Sometimes chronic illness, stress, or overuse of caffeine can lead to an imbalance or deficiency of calcium.

- Potassium deficiency can be a significant problem for older people. It is characterized by muscular weakness, disorientation, depression, and irritability. This deficiency becomes more common with age, especially among people who are on diuretics or who have had prolonged diarrhea. You can reestablish a balance in your diet by eating dried fruits, apricots, oranges, grapefruit, potatoes, dried peas, beans, peanut butter, bananas, and apple juice—all of which are good sources of potassium.

A Sad Report on Bad Nutrition

The hazards of poor nutrition and its relationship to disease are painfully clear when you look at a number of medical histories. In the case of "Dora Solomon," her diet, her lack of exercise, and the stress in her life turned poor health into personal disaster.

Dora, an attractive five-foot-seven-inch woman, went through menopause at the age of fifty. With the onset of menopause, her body lost estrogen, which she didn't replace. That same year, her husband had a stroke and was partially disabled. He was ill for the next twelve years, until his death. During the years after his stroke, he stayed on a low-cholesterol diet, which meant high protein with no milk or dairy products; Dora followed the same diet as her husband and ate no dairy products at a time when she should have increased her intake of calcium to at least one hundred milligrams a day because of her age. Like her husband, Dora was a big coffee drinker—and as we've learned, calcium absorption is hampered by caffeine.

In addition, from the age of fifty to sixty-two, Dora led an extraordinarily sedentary life. Before that, she had had little exercise, but now she had almost none. With the exception of weekly trips to the grocery store, she moved around very little. Mainly, she sat and read or watched television with her husband.

At the age of sixty, Dora developed a puffiness and itchiness around her eyes. She went to the dermatologist, who didn't know what it was but prescribed cortisone orally. She took the cortisone over several weeks. When the puffiness subsided, she stopped the pills. When it started again, she began taking her remaining pills *without asking the doctor about it*. She had not been told that this medication is dangerous and must be taken in specific dosages. Nor had she been told that you can't stop this medication suddenly; you have to be withdrawn gradually.

A long period of decline in her health followed. She

visited a number of doctors but never found out what
was the matter with her. Eventually, she fell down and
broke her pelvis. She was hospitalized and diagnosed
as having a very bad case of osteoporosis. When more
sophisticated tests were taken, Cushing's syndrome was
also diagnosed. The tumors caused the adrenals to pump
excess natural body cortisone into the body, which
caused bone destruction and added, of course, to all the
other primary conspiring elements—calcium loss, estrogen loss, and lack of weight-bearing exercise—that
contributed to her osteoporosis. Altogether, Dora lost
eight inches in height from fractured vertebrae, a result
of the osteoporosis. She is now seventy-four and basically moves only from one chair to another. Her spirits
and outlook on life are dim. It's not farfetched to spec-
ulate that with a proper diet that included calcium and
a half-hour walk a day accompanied by the medical
option of estrogen replacement, Dora Solomon would
be much better off today. She would still have Cushing's, but with regular medical care and an earlier diagnosis, she wouldn't have experienced such dire
consequences.

A Good Report on Balancing Your Nutrition

Just as the ill effects can be seen from one's nutritional
intake, so the good effects can also be seen and measured. In contrast to Dora's sad story, there is her
brother-in-law's happy one. "Edward Fox," who married Dora's sister, Louise, had a slight heart attack when
he was fifty-eight. Following his crisis, he changed his
diet and his life-style. Now, at the age of seventy-eight,
he and his seventy-two-year-old wife, Louise, play tennis every morning for at least an hour and a half. After
their game, they return home to have a breakfast of bran
cereal, whole wheat toast, jam, cheese, juice, and coffee. They don't eat anything else (except an occasional
piece of fruit) until dinnertime, when Edward has a
before-dinner drink (which he's been having for at least

fifty years), and then they eat meat, fish, or poultry, vegetables, salad, and wine.

If you have any nutrient deficiencies, most likely you can correct them with a good diet and the use of appropriate food supplements. According to Dr. Jeffrey Blumberg, studies over the past twenty years have provided clear evidence that immune function that has been impaired by specific nutrient deficiencies can be restored if those deficiencies are repaired. Even more promising is research at Tufts University and at other gerontological centers that continues to look for answers as to whether, by appropriate nutritional maintenance, the immune system can be fortified up to keep it "young."

Some progress is being made. In his work with laboratory animals, for instance, Dr. Blumberg found that Vitamin E has a stimulating effect on old mice with "old" immune systems. Given high levels of Vitamin E for relatively short periods of time, the immune systems of these animals become as vigorous as the immune systems of young mice. If the same holds true in humans, high doses of Vitamin E and other vitamins may eventually be found to invigorate the immune systems of older people and slow down the incidence of infectious diseases.

At the University of California at Los Angeles, Dr. Roy Wolford, who heads the research laboratory for the study of immunology and the aging process, cites evidence that "undernutrition without malnutrition" has slowed down the rate of aging and extended the maximum life span of laboratory mice. Dr. Wolford believes that this research indicates that eating less, but eating well, gives us credible prospects not only for staying healthy by building up the immune system, but also for extending the maximum life span perhaps by two or three decades beyond what it is today.

In his book *Maximum Life Span*, Dr. Wolford says that information is already available to enable us to live to be more than 120 years old if we begin early enough and adhere religiously to a lifelong regimen of dietary restriction. For undernutrition to work without a person becoming malnourished, however, Dr. Wolford adds that food intake must be balanced, high in fiber content, and reasonably low in sodium. Dr. Wolford reveals that he personally fasts two days out of seven and eats a nutritious, supplemented diet the other five days. He runs twelve miles and swims one to two miles per week. He takes daily food supplements in divided doses, including vitamin E (600 IU); selenium (160 micrograms); BHT (250 milligrams); Cysteine (300 milligrams); methionine (120 milligrams); Ascorbyl palmitate (600 milligrams); vitamin C (1000 milligrams); and bioflavinoids (300 milligrams).

Changing Your Habits Affects Your Medications

If you change your diet, it may have an effect on medications that you are taking for chronic conditions. When Joe Lepore had a stroke a few years ago, for instance, he was put on blood pressure pills. His daughter, Cynthia Rivelli, helped him change his diet by beginning to cook salt-free foods for him when she visited him in the country on weekends. Pretty soon he was cooking all his food without salt, and enjoying it. Then suddenly he got sick.

"Dad got really sick, and it turned out it was because of the blood pressure pills he was taking," says Cynthia. "He had lowered his blood pressure by changing his diet, but he was still taking his blood pressure pills. He was also taking medication for gout that he should have been taking only when he needed it."

Now he takes no heart medication, aspirin, or anything else on a regular basis. Every now and then, he takes a gout pill. He works in his garden every day, takes long walks, and during hunting and fishing seasons, he's out with his gun or his fishing rod for long and often productive days.

The moral of Joe's story is twofold. First is that a change in your diet can eliminate your need for pills. Second is that if you change your diet, tell your doctor about it. Ask him to check you out. If you're lucky, you may not need your pills anymore—or if you do need them, the dosage may change.

ANOTHER PROVEN PATH: THE BENEFITS OF EXERCISE

Many gerontologists believe that in addition to good nutrition, exercise is a critical factor in staying "young" and healthy as you age. Many say that exercise may be the single most effective way to slow down aging and lengthen life.

The benefits of exercise aren't a figment of the imagination. In studying the life-styles and habits of more than a million people over twenty years' time, the American Cancer Society found that death rates were significantly higher among people who did not exercise. As exercise increased, mortality rates dropped.

"If exercise could be packed into a pill," says Dr. Butler at Mount Sinai Medical Center, "it would be the single most widely prescribed and beneficial medicine in the nation."

Researchers tell us that a change from a sedentary life-style to one of moderate but regular exercise can be an overall aid to health. In fact, they may eventually find out that exercise is a major factor in keeping the immune system healthy, allowing the body to maintain, repair, and improve itself on a long-term basis. Currently, however, according to Dr. Maria Fiatarone, a physician in the Division of Gerontology at Harvard Medical School, there's no direct experimental evidence of the long-term effect of exercise on the immune system of older people. But there is evidence, she says, that a bout of exercise stimulates natural killer cells.

These cells are thought to be important in killing cells infected with viruses and in suppressing the growth and spread of cancer cells.

Dr. Fiatarone and her colleagues conducted an experiment in which blood samples were taken from older people before and after they rode stationary bicycles an average of twelve minutes. She found that after the exercise, hormones secreted by white blood cells that stimulate the immune system were activated.

"We don't know what long-term effect this could have on the immune system of older people," she said, "but we hope eventually to find out. The only study that demonstrated a long-lasting effect of exercise on the immune system showed that athletes who had trained over a period of time had a higher-than-normal level of this hormone that stimulates the immune system."

Research from the National Institute on Aging suggests that regular exercise can strengthen your heart and lungs, lower your blood pressure, and protect you against the start of adult-onset diabetes. If you are already diabetic, it can reduce your need for insulin, lower your blood-sugar levels, and improve your glucose tolerance. Among other things, it also stimulates healthy circulation of the blood and aids in both digestion and elimination. It can strengthen and tone your muscles and help you move more easily by keeping your joints, tendons, and ligaments more flexible.

Exercise for women is particularly important since it helps build bone mass and prevent osteoporosis. Vigorous physical exercise is now the only non-pharmacological means of building up bone after normal bone growth is completed. Recent studies have shown that older women can build up their bone mass even if they start exercising late in life.

Exercise is also extremely helpful in preventing cardiovascular disease. Dr. Butler points out that a considerable number of coronary arteriosclerotic deaths in the

United States are eminently preventable by changes in life-style that include exercise.

Recently I talked with "Minerva Easton," a seventy-eight-year-old who had just emerged from the swimming pool at the YMCA in Princeton, New Jersey, where she goes to swim three times a week as part of a hydro-aerobics class for senior citizens. "I'll tell you, since I started this, I'm in better shape," she said, shaking water out of her curly gray hair. "I know it's good for my heart and my muscles, but the bigger thing is that it makes me *feel* great. My friends over there will tell you the same thing. This may be good for the body, but what it does for the spirit is far more important."

Clearly, a major benefit of exercise is the sense of well-being you get from it. There's a physiological basis suggested for the good spirits, in that the brain releases natural opiatelike substances called endorphins, which may induce that sense of well-being. Activity naturally gives you more energy as well. Even if you feel tired when you start, the flow of oxygen and blood and endorphins seems to lift that feeling of tiredness and help you avoid fatigue. Because exercise makes you less tense, it also makes you look better. The spin-off is that your appearance improves along with your self-confidence.

A Prescription for Exercise

If you don't exercise now, you may want to start. Consult your doctor about your condition, your plan, and any precautions you should take. If you don't know where to start, your local YMCA may be a good place to begin. Most YMCAs and YWCAs have programs that range from light aerobic exercise classes to swim groups to dance lessons or the Chinese form of exercise, t'ai chi ch'uan. Some specific fitness classes for "seniors" focus on flexibility and key muscle groups and are aimed at getting older people in shape.

Aerobic exercise, which gives your cardiovascular system the workout it needs, is said to be the most effective form of exercise. This kind of exercise uses the large muscle groups of your body in rhythmical and continuous movement for prolonged periods of time. It causes the pulse rate to reach 80 percent of its maximum for at least a twenty-minute period, and helps the body to take in, transport, and use more oxygen at an increased rate. Good and available forms of aerobic exercise include swimming, jogging, fast walking, calisthenics, rowing, and bicycling.

Sometimes good hard work in your yard gives you the fresh air and the exercise you need. Henry Quigley, who's seventy-three, told me about his ninety-four-year-old mother's daily fare:

"Ida Murray, she doesn't take nothing. No pills. She still lives in her own house and she still works in her yard. You wouldn't believe the way she works! Up to this year, she mowed her own lawn. She wouldn't let us do nothing. This year we finally convinced her to let someone else mow it. This year she had corn, potatoes, beans, cucumbers, and tomatoes in her garden.

"She'll get out in the heat of day and weed and work. . . . We try to convince her to work early in the morning and late in the day to avoid the sun, but she goes out when she wants to in the heat of the day. The neighbors say to us, 'Someday you're going to come up here and your mother's going to be dead, lying in the garden.' Ida says, 'Well, if that's where I am when I go, I'd go happy.' "

Many people sixty-five and older enjoy tennis, racquetball, golf, baseball, fencing, skiing, and hiking. There is also modified aerobic dance, yoga, and exercise that involves warm-ups, stretches, and calisthenics. Bowling, bird walks, badminton, volleyball, or going out dancing are also good forms of exercise.

You may enjoy exercising at home to a record or a videotape, either by yourself or with friends. Or you may decide to start with short walks and then extend those walks.

If you like company, most communities have centers where people sixty-five and older can join exercise classes and other recreational programs. Look into your local newspaper for ideas. Call your local church or synagogue, your senior citizens' center, or the local park or recreation center to find out what's available. It may be the best preventative medicine you'll ever take.

Not exercising is to invite trouble with stiffness, physical discomfort, and poor circulation. Even if you are in a wheelchair, you can still do exercises to improve your strength and sense of well-being. Toe lifts, leg lifts, arm stretches, and rotating your head to the left and right and up and down can help your circulation and keep your muscles healthier.

"A prescription for physical activity or exercise is as important as any prescription for medication," says Lawrence J. Frankel and Betty Byrd Richard in their book, *Be Alive As Long As You Live*. "You invite weariness and boredom, physical discomfort, depression, and even death when you do not motivate yourself to be physically and mentally active to the limit of your ability. To live effectively, with real purpose, and not merely to exist, you must be active.

"Your own body is the one machine that breaks down when *not* used; it works better, unquestionably, the more you use it."

If you've been leading a sedentary life and you want to become active, ask your doctor if there are any kinds of exercises you should avoid. Certainly, if you have any health problems or you're at all doubtful about what to do, consult your physician. Some people feel they should have a complete physical, and this may well be recommended in your case. According to Per-Olaf Astrand and Kaare Rodahl, authors of *Textbook of Work Physiology*, however, if there's a question of whether to exercise or not to exercise, exercise should always win out. "In principle, there is less risk in activity than in inactivity," says Drs. Astrand and Rodahl. "Our opinion is that it is more advisable to pass a careful medical examination if one intends to be sedentary in order to establish whether one's state of health is good enough to stand the inactivity."

Take It Easy

The American Association of Retired Persons suggests that it's always important to warm up by walking or stretching before you start exercising. The experience is more gentle for the body if you gradually increase the intensity until your pulse rate, respiration rate, and body temperature are elevated. They suggest that once you have begun your daily exercise program, you keep the following pointers in mind:

- Start gradually, about five to ten minutes at first.
- Increase the amount of exercise each day, up to about twenty-five minutes.
- Avoid dizziness by pausing briefly before changing direction.
- Breathe deeply and evenly between exercises and during exercise. Don't hold your breath.
- Rest whenever necessary.
- Keep a daily written record of your progress.
- Exercise to lively music, TV, or with friends for added enjoyment.
- Make exercising a part of your daily routine.

LAUGHTER, TOUCHING, AND ATTITUDE

Evidence has been accumulating in medical centers across the country that the mind has a far more dramatic effect on our bodies than scientists have believed. Greater understanding of the chemistry of the brain has led researchers to discover that our feelings of joy, grief, and contentment are linked to our physiological resistance to sickness and disease. There are signs that using relaxation techniques such as yoga, meditation, and biofeedback may actually have the power to diminish pain and strengthen the immune system to resist many kinds of illnesses.

"I believe that as you get older, the body doesn't function because of use, misuse, and lack of use," says Jaki Jackson, a yoga teacher in East Hampton, New York, who often teaches classes to older people at the senior citizens' center. "I try to get older people to tell me what they want for themselves, not what they don't want. I don't want to hear, 'My knee can't bend.' I want to hear, 'I want to bend my knees.' Language has a lot to do with how we live. What we think and talk about is what we create for ourselves.

"I think that one way to keep our health as we get older is to diversify our habits, perform tasks differently. If you're used to putting your right foot forward first, put your left foot forward instead. Subject yourself to change.

"I believe in laughing. It changes you physiologically. It utilizes a whole different set of muscles. It exercises your stomach and your belly, making your intestines and your diaphragm move. A good belly laugh convulses your whole system. It loosens the muscles in your face and often brings tears to your eyes.

"Basically, laughter is a form of a physical workout. I'd consider it a necessary tool for staying in shape.

"Part of the problem is that as you get older, you're not exploring your physical body as much. Other people aren't touching your body as much—and you need physical contact. You need the stimulation for your brain, for your skin, for your lymph system. The elderly aren't fragile and untouchable. They need the touching to keep the flow going, to keep the circuits connected.

"All of us can stay mentally alert and vital, and physically young as well. I've known an eighty-four-year-old who played an excellent game of tennis. He could go out and play two great sets and still beat the younger players. My friend Anna's husband dives for clams and still does construction work, and he's seventy-nine. Exercise is one thing, but awareness, new perceptions, and the flexibility to keep moving and reorganizing on a higher level are what keep you young."

The Benefits of Relaxation

Most people can remember, when they're tense, how much better they feel when they're relaxed. New research is showing that deep relaxation practiced regularly may decrease the body's susceptibility to disease and produce other medically valuable physiological changes. In 1984, the National Institute of Health recommended the use of relaxation techniques, along with salt restriction and weight loss, as the first therapy for mild hypertension, before the use of medication.

Deep relaxation releases muscle tension, lowers blood pressure, and slows the heart and breathing rates. Although relaxing activities help, the kind of relaxation that achieves physiological results involves a technique that breaks the train of everyday thought and decreases the activity of the central nervous system.

In many patients with chronic, unbearable pain, deep-relaxation training has brought significant relief from severe pain arising from backache, chronic migraine or tension headaches, and pain from diseases such as cancer. Asthmatics can widen their restricted respiratory passages when they relax deeply as well as reduce the emotional upsets that often trigger attacks. Diabetics can reduce their need for insulin, according to recent reports, because relaxation improves the body's ability to regulate glucose.

In research conducted at Harvard Medical School in

Boston, relaxation alone was found to increase defenses against upper-respiratory infections. According to a report in *Health Psychology*, Ohio State researchers taught relaxation techniques to residents of a retirement home, whose average age was seventy-four. After a month of training, their levels of natural killer cells and antibodies—indicators of resistance to tumors and viruses—had improved significantly.

If you have trouble relaxing, or if you want to lower your stress levels and strengthen your resistance to disease, you may want to explore yoga classes, various forms of meditation, hypnosis, or biofeedback.

Attitude Makes a Difference

Many of the older people I talked with said that, in their experience, what really worked when it came to living a long and healthy life was *attitude*. They felt that having a sense of adventure and optimism—a positive attitude—was probably more important than any other single factor they could name.

They are right. Several recent studies have confirmed that people's own evaluation of their health is the best predictor of who will live or die over the next decade. If people say their health is "excellent," they are seven times less likely to die in the next twelve years than people who say their health is "poor," according to a long-term study by the Federal Public Health Service. People's attitudes and estimates about their health and well-being outperformed even physical examinations as long-term predictors of their mortality.

"If you just sit around and complain about all the things that are wrong all the time, you aren't that alive anyway," says Joy Sorenson, an eighty-one-year-old in Los Angeles, California. "I know we all like to compare our aches and pains sometimes, but that's just entertainment. What's really important to my health, I know is my attitude. No sickness has been that big to me, even though I've had a couple of serious rounds. I walk and I eat well, but I do those things because I want to and because I care. That's attitude for you. It comes before anything else.''

C H A P T E R   12

★

Working on Your Own Behalf—
Helping Your Doctors Help You

It is nine years now since I met Mr. MacGregor, in the neurology clinic of St. Dunstan's, an old-people's home where I once worked, but I remember him—I see him—as if it were yesterday.

"What's the problem?" I asked, as he tilted in.

"Problem? No problem—none that I know of . . . But others keep telling me I lean to the side: 'You're like the Leaning Tower of Pisa,' they say. 'A bit more tilt, and you'll topple right over.' "

"But *you* don't feel any tilt?"

"I feel fine. I don't know what they mean. How *could* I be tilted without knowing I was?"

"It sounds a queer business," I agreed. "Let's have a look. I'd like to see you stand and take a little stroll—just from here to that wall and back. I want to see for myself, *and I want you to see, too*. We'll take a videotape of you walking and play it right back."

"Suits me, Doc," he said, and, after a couple of lunges, stood up. What a fine old chap, I thought. Ninety-three—and he doesn't look a day past seventy. Alert, bright as a button. Good for a hundred. And strong as a coal-heaver, even if he does have Parkinson's disease. He was walking, now, confidently, swiftly, but canted over, improbably, a good twenty degrees, his centre of gravity way off to the left, maintaining his balance by the narrowest possible margin.

"There!" he said with a pleased smile. "See! No problems—I walked straight as a die."

"Did you, indeed, Mr. MacGregor?" I asked. "I want you to judge for yourself."

I rewound the tape and played it back. He was profoundly shocked when he saw himself on the screen. His eyes bulged, his jaw dropped, and he muttered, "I'll be damned!" And then, "They're right, I *am* over to one side. I *see* it here clear enough, but I've no sense of it. I don't *feel* it."

"That's it," I said. "That's the heart of the problem."

from *The Man Who Mistook His Wife for a Hat and Other Clinical Tales*, by Oliver Sacks

In selecting your doctor—whether it's an internist, a physician's assistant, an osteopath, a dentist, a cardiac specialist, or an eye doctor—it's very important to select a person whose judgment you trust, and who is willing, like Dr. Sacks, to spend time addressing your concerns. Even when your doctor's credentials are impeccable, it's important to trust that this person will listen to you, give you the time to hear what's important to you, care about how you feel, and respect your wish to function well in your life. It's important to have a doctor who makes sense to you and who is willing to discuss your condition and your treatment alternatives with you if you are sick. It may be that you're the type of person who, if faced with a medical problem, wants your doctor to make all the decisions for you. If so, then find a doctor whom you trust to make good decisions for you. If so, then find a doctor whom you trust to make good decisions on your behalf. If you want to understand your options and participate in your own healing process, make sure you find a doctor who will discuss the risks and benefits of various treatments and suggest alternative methods of making your condition better—without medication—when it is appropriate.

Remember that your physician's medical knowledge and judgment are based in large part on probabilities and uncertainties. Your doctor has value systems and personal psychology that affect his or her decisions in a subjective way. Dr. Constance Molino Park, at Columbia Presbyterian Medical Center in New York City, points out that when faced with uncertainty, physicians whose personal psychology is more consistent with "man controlling his destiny" (interventionist physicians) will probably present risky procedures in a more positive light than physicians who tend to believe more in "watchful waiting" (conservative physicians). Furthermore, the doctor's fear of his own vulnerability, says Dr. Park, can present an emotional barrier to the open and effective disclosure of information that would promote discussion of pain, suffering, and death.

Since your doctor's clinical decisions regarding your health are apt to involve many complex factors, there's often no one "correct" path to take. If you are ill, your clarity is knowing what risks you're willing to take and what discomforts you're willing to live with will be important considerations in choosing a course of treatment that will work for you. A doctor who is aware of your life-style, concerns, socioeconomic conditions, and stresses will also be able to help you make the life-style adaptations that are often required by chronic diseases or multiple conditions.

Usually when you first meet a doctor, you go into his or her waiting room with an expectation, often a hope, of what kind of experience and what kind of person you'll encounter there. This is part of what you transfer to your doctor when you first meet him or her.

"Some patients look for someone to solve all their problems," says Nancy S. Foldi, Ph.D., a clinical neuropsychologist at the Coffey Geriatric Clinic at Mount Sinai Medical Center. "Others may view the doctor in a negative or confronting way. They're hardly eager to sit through another visit, and even assume, ahead of time, that it will be a waste of time." Thus, how a person imagines the visit can influence how the actual visit transpires, largely because of these expectations.

"Often, the way you view yourself with your doctor is not unlike the way you view yourself with other people," says Dr. Foldi. "If someone sees the doctor as knowing everything and himself as knowing nothing, or if someone uses an abrupt style with the doctor, it may occur that the person mirrors that style in other relationships, professional or otherwise. It is worth a moment's thought to consider what your feelings and expectations are when you're about to meet a new team or doctor, or even to think about how you've interacted with doctors before. The doctor-patient relationship is a two-way street that both parties have to work at, and it's worth a try not to let prior expectations get in the way of a realistic rapport."

A JOINT RESPONSIBILITY

The first requirement of good medicine is the doctor-patient relationship. This relationship should be one of mutual understanding, respect, and trust. The treatment process is going on between you and your doctor. There's no magic to the physician's treatment plan. It's a dynamic process that requires your active participation. As we've pointed out before, studies have established that communications between patients and their doctors about their medications are inadequate. More than a third of patients over sixty-five say they leave their doctor's office with no information about the drugs prescribed to them. The majority of older patients also report that they don't receive information from their physicians about why they're taking the medications, how to take them, or what side effects or contraindications they should expect. They get incomplete or confusing instructions. Patients also report that in addition to not being given answers, *they don't ask questions*.

This problem is shared by both physician and patient. "Sometimes the patient and the physician have hang-ups about aging, disability, disfigurement, and death that prevent rapport and good communication," says Dr. Robert N. Butler, in *The Geriatric Patient*. "I have had opportunities to observe good and bad doctor-patient relationships. For the lonely and worried patient, I have no doubt that simply being seen and heard by a trusted physician has a therapeutic effect; the patient may still have heart disease or cancer, but his or her morale is uplifted and the encounter promotes ability to function. When trust and respect are lacking on either side of the consulting desk, the results can be disastrous: instead of making the most of the patient's abilities, the relationship becomes an obstacle to effective clinical treatment."

Communication is vital. You can't afford to wait for the doctor to provide you with all the answers. Nor can you assume the doctor is able to read your mind. You have to ask questions, follow up on tests, ask about results. The results of noncommunication can leave you, at the least, with a lack of ease. At worst, the results of miscommunication or noncommunication over serious medical issues an be fatal.

Attitudes that Get in the Way
The attitude that the doctor is not to be bothered, and that his authority should not be questioned, can be a dangerous one—particularly if it leads to your withholding important information. If you assume the doctor knows all the answers, even when you haven't asked the questions, you may find yourself in deep trouble. Additionally, this attitude can make you feel more help-

less—which doesn't add to your spirit of health and determination to recover or to stay well. Some older people with whom I talked don't even ask the doctor to tell them what he thinks is wrong with them. They come into the doctor's office prepared to accept totally whatever the doctor says—no matter what it is. Being sick makes this regression more likely. If you take on this passive attitude, however, you'll probably find yourself with questions in the middle of the night and a treatment plan that may fail to work.

Doctor as Deity

"When our children were little, we all thought the doctor was God," says case worker Elaine Johannes, who works with people over sixty who have difficult problems that range from Medicare insurance to where to live or where to buy generic drugs. "Younger people have exploded that myth, but the older generation still holds it to a large extent.

"Most people have an attitude that the doctor knows everything about every possible disease, the consequences of the condition, medicines, and prices. They even think the doctor understands Medicare and their medical costs, but he or she usually doesn't.

"Basically, you have to be a very strong person to argue with your doctor. Urban people have more choices and are more willing to question. Rural people say, 'We don't dare question. There's only one physician and one hospital here that can care for me.' They don't want to jeopardize their care by antagonizing their doctor or their hospital.

"Sometimes if an older person asks a question and the doctor doesn't know the answer, he'll say, 'That's not important.' Then the older person is crushed because he feels stupid. He got up his nerve to ask and then the doctor shoots him down."

At other times, patients feel they don't dare "impose" on their doctor with their questions. It's not unheard of for an older person who feels sick from medications not to tell the doctor because of a fear that the doctor will feel badly because the treatment didn't work. They also avoid telling him that they visited another doctor and that the other doctor gave them medication. Or, if they're interested in a second opinion, they may not feel that they should say so because it would insult him.

" 'I don't want to hurt his feelings,' or 'I don't want to make him angry' are common reasons older people, women particularly, give for not reporting back to their doctors,'' says geriatric nurse Sylvia McBurnie. ''They need to learn that it's okay to tell the doctor when they haven't been feeling well. They need to know that in fact, their telling the doctor helps him because it opens up dialogue and provides the doctor with information he needs.

''Some doctors don't remember to ask whether you have allergies or strange reactions to medications,'' says Ms. McBurnie, ''so it's your responsibility as a consumer to inform them of your allergies and your other medications. It's your right and your responsibility to ask questions about your condition and your medicines. You *must* tell your doctor when you're seeing other doctors and getting medications from them.''

Get Your Answers
''Bring up things with your doctor, and ask questions,'' says pharmacist and consultant Randall Wright. ''In all my years, I only heard of two physicians who blew up when they were asked questions by pharmacists. They were insecure. Most doctors will explain their reasons.

''As a rule, doctors are secure, smart people. They'll say, 'Yes, go ahead, ask. Get a second opinion. It makes me look good.' Having an opinion confirmed makes them feel better and it makes the patients feel better.''

Many doctors themselves are critical of the concept of doctor as deity. ''We have to get away from the autocratic, dictatorial doctor-patient relationship," says Dr. Butler. "You must remember that doctors are your servants! You pay them! They're not kings and queens!"

Dr. Tom Reynolds, a physician in Albany, New York, who used to work at Memorial Sloan-Kettering Cancer Center in New York City, put it differently. "There's only one valid way for patients to look at us," he said during a recent interview. "We're providing a service. We're just like hairdressers—we're there to make people feel better. You know how a woman goes to a hairdresser, gets her hair done, and feels better? We doctors should make her feel the same way. It may be that we have more of an effect on the overall quality of our patients' lives, but in terms of importance, we're no different from hairdressers. Surgeons are no different from the people who cut and sew material to make clothes."

Perhaps partially in reaction to the status and authority of doctors, some people remain silent—not because they think of their physicians as gods, they say, but because they think that if doctors are going to charge so much, they shouldn't have to "earn their nickel" by "proving" what they know.

"He didn't tell me anything I didn't already know," "Sarah Borchardt" said a friend told her recently after a trip to the doctor. "You'd think he's so smart, being a doctor."

"Well, did you tell him that you've been feeling dizzy when you stand up?"

"No."

"Did you tell him about the stomachaches?"

"No, he ought to tell me, not the other way around! What does he charge all that money for?!"

DOCTORS AS FARMERS AND MIDWIVES

The doctor-patient relationship has changed a great deal
within the lifetime of people in their sixties, seventies,
eighties, and nineties. As sociologist Paul Starr docu-
ments in his informative book, *The Social Transformation of American Medicine*, the authority of the
medical profession increased dramatically during the
first few decades of this century.

Prior to that, particularly in the early 1800s in this
country, doctors didn't have the wealth, status, or authority they gained after 1910. They weren't automatically endowed with public respect. "The doctor was
more a courier than an autocrat," Dr. Starr writes.
Many doctors couldn't support themselves merely from
their practice. They had to farm or hold extra jobs—
from pulling teeth to looking after farmers' livestock to
working as pharmacists or midwives. Unlike the standards of today, when doctors are required to go through
four years of liberal arts training, four years of medical
school, and four years of supervised hospital training,
as well as passing standardized tests to get into medical
school, to graduate from medical school, and to qualify
as certified specialists, physicians in those days had no
fixed career patterns. They might or might not have
gone to medical school and might or might not have
served an apprenticeship. Dr. Starr points out that just
as the patient had no guarantee of his doctor's training
or reliable, measurable technical skills, the physician
had no certainty of social and economic rewards.

The growth of medical authority, related to the success of science, is revolutionizing other aspects of medicine as well as creating pervasive changes in everyday
experience. Dr. Starr explains how the new diagnostic
technologies at the disposal of physicians gave them
increased power. With the stethoscope, doctors could
hear something the patient couldn't hear. Their powers
expanded with the microscope, with X rays, with chem-

ical and bacteriological tests for disease. With this new apparatus for medical measurement, they could also simultaneously review and discuss what they saw with their colleagues—which strengthened their ability for objective judgment. People began increasingly to resort to professional advice for interpretations of the new conditions of life. Their perceptions of the value of specialized knowledge were also altered by the pervasive changes in normal life that had been brought about by revolutions in technology and social change. People's waning belief in their own ability to understand the world without higher education or training increased their reliance on professionals and enhanced the authority of professional medicine.

A Turning of the Wheel

Now, once again, the authority of the medical professional is undergoing a process of change. In the past twenty years, the medical profession has been heavily criticized, and a "crisis in health care" that has to do with the cost and availability of services has become the focus of active concern and legislation. A new emphasis on patients' rights to health care, and their rights within that care, have changed, with a growing awareness on the part of consumers everywhere. Certainly, there's a great deal of ambivalence when it comes to the authority of the medical community these days. At its most extreme, the new view is that patients must be protected from their doctors, while a milder form is the conviction that, as consumers, patients should exercise their rights to require informed consent, their right to refuse treatment, their right to see their own medical records, and their right to participate in therapeutic decisions. There is also a change in that doctors and hospitals are sharing more information and authority with their patients.

HELP THEM HELP YOU

The very circumstances of sickness promote dependency and your acceptance of the doctor's judgment. When you're in pain, or feel fearful and uncomfortable, you want to be reassured and taken care of. In most cases when you are under the care of a good physician, this dependency is valuable. Your willingness to cooperate and do what the doctor tells you to do is important to the success of your treatment. Certainly, you don't have the doctor's expertise, and when you're very sick, you're often in no position to judge your own needs. Even doctors go to other physicians rather than treat themselves, a practice based on the old maxim that a doctor who treats himself has a fool for a patient and a knave for a doctor.

Obviously, in critical, emergency situations, moment-to-moment decisions must be turned over entirely to your doctor. You can't monitor complex serum levels or make decisions about titration, dehydration, or intravenous feedings. You're not trained in reading charts, evaluating an electrocardiogram, or deciding which antibiotic would be most effective. Aside from their specialized knowledge of your medical condition, doctors have an advantage in making judgments about what will serve you best. This is their work.

You, however, can help doctors make the most of what they do if you're alert to what's happening to you. "Paul Howe," for instance, was getting an emergency blood transfusion his doctor had ordered, and he intervened effectively on his own behalf. "I was on the blood by nine o'clock," Paul said later from his home in Denver, Colorado, "and by about a quarter of twelve I dropped off to sleep for five minutes. I woke up with my teeth chattering and I was shaking all over from a chill that was uncontrollable. I was gasping for breath and gagging. The nurse was ready to shoot me with a diuretic and then to start the next unit of blood.

"There were two nurses there by that time. I said, 'I'll be dead in ten minutes if you do the wrong thing. Call the doctor and tell him to stop the transfusion, have him authorize Tylenol to quiet me, and see whether or not he wants me to have the diuretic or any more blood under this condition.' "

The nurse called the doctor, who said to stop the transfusions and to give Paul the diuretic and the Tylenol. Almost instantly after the transfusion had been stopped and the diuretic injected, Paul's breathing eased and his body warmed. In less than five minutes he was urinating and continued to urinate every three to five minutes for the next hour. He had been nearly drowning in the liquid that had built up in his lungs from the fluids that had drained into his body tissues from the transfusion. Even though he hadn't known what to do himself, he knew how to ask for the help he needed. He knew that Tylenol might help quiet his nerves, and he suggested it. As it turned out, he was right.

Even in emergency situations, you can ask intelligent questions and learn what the doctor is doing for you. You can find out ways to comply with treatment and become aware of what's happening to you. If you're in the hospital, for instance, and the doctor tells you you're going to be given a certain medication at 6:00 P.M., and it's still not there by 8:00 P.M., you can find out why it has not been given to you. If you have not received it by 10:00 P.M., call your doctor. Your alertness and your compliance with the doctor's well-informed judgments can make all the difference in your physician's ability to help you.

If you are one of those "humbled parties" who are afraid to speak up when they meet with doctors, then perhaps it's time to equalize the relationships. Of course you don't have your doctor's technical expertise or judgment, but you are the person living in your body and you should understand what you're doing for it and why. You need to approach your doctor with as assertive an attitude on your own behalf as you would take on behalf of your friend of your child.

Certainly, when you understand your treatment and medication, it's much easier to comply with what your doctor wants you to do. Remember that ultimately the decisions are yours, as is the responsibility. If you don't like the way you feel on a particular medicine, say so. Don't be shy. Ask the doctor about alternative methods or medications.

Understanding Your Choices

Dr. Diane Meier, chief of the Coffey Geriatric Center at Mount Sinai Hospital, says she finds that the majority of her patients understand that it's their responsibility to take their medicines or not, to follow their exercise programs or not, and to make dietary changes or not. "It's the patients' responsibility to choose what to do," she says, "and they know I respect that choice."

In one case, for instance, Dr. Meier recommended that an eighty-two-year-old patient of hers with a persistent cough have a bronchoscopy, an uncomfortable and sometimes dangerous procedure in which a flexible tube containing glass fibers with special optical properties is put down the throat. The light from the glass fibers returns a clear magnified image from the end of the tube so that the doctors can take a look inside the throat. Her patient thought about it and said, "I don't want it." Dr. Meier said, "Okay, it's your decision."

"I respect her decision," she said, talking about the case later. "She knows what's acceptable to her. Her life is marginally pleasurable to her as it is, and she's not willing to make it that much less pleasurable in order to possibly live longer.

"On the other hand, I have another patient who's eighty-nine and lives alone with her husband and functions very well. Her right hand is nonfunctional and she's had several major health problems, but she's happy with her life and she gets every procedure that she'd get if she were forty years younger. She wants to live and she wants optimal health conditions while she's at it. The perspective differs with the patient, and my approach differs accordingly."

As Dr. Meier pointed out, you're likely to make specific knotty medical decisions on the basis of what matters to you in your life. If, as we've said, your sex life matters to you, you won't want to undergo certain procedures or take certain medications that are known absolutely to adversely affect your sexual drive or performance. If your day-to-day comfort is barely acceptable to you the way it is, you may not want to risk certain diagnostic procedures that could cause you more pain and discomfort. You may have strong feelings that if you are terminally ill, you do or do not want drastic measures taken when your heart stops beating or you go into a coma. If you have a condition that is gradually worsening and you know, for instance, that you may die within a certain period of time, you may want to talk with your family and your doctor about what procedures you want. Agreeing on these matters ahead of time can make the eventual medical crisis as easy as possible on all of you. Letting your family know what you want done can relieve them of the responsibility of making decisions for you.

Discussing all these important personal issues and making decisions based on your wishes and the informed judgments of your doctor can be extremely rewarding. Often it provides an opportunity to air big fears that otherwise might be ignored. Acknowledging them can be a big relief. As Dr. Meier said one day during a team meeting at the geriatric clinic, "Just in terms of how we write things up on the workup sheet, medical issues are on the top, and social issues are at the bottom. It's usually not in that sequence for the patient."

Always make sure you understand the terms of your gamble. If your choice is a drug or a procedure that

will extend your life by three years but leave you unable
to speak, you've got to decide what matters to you most.
You need to know as much as possible to evaluate and
decide whether you're willing to take those risks. Some
drugs are so lethal that they're only prescribed for very
serious illnesses. If your doctor prescribes one of these
to you—whether it's for cancer, your heart, or whatever—make sure he fully explains the risks to you. Remember, it's your choice, not your doctor's. Don't
hesitate to take the time you need to make your decision.

In light of the kinds of issues you may want or need
to discuss with your doctors—from medication problems to your philosophy regarding what to do about life-
support systems—it's extremely important that you have
a physician who respects your standards and priorities
and the quality of life you want to preserve.

EVALUATE YOUR DOCTOR'S ATTITUDE

A doctor's attitude that you're a bumbling old goat
makes good communication nearly impossible. The
doctors who condescend to you, who don't answer your
questions or don't exhibit an interest in your situation,
aren't worth your time or the expense involved in seeing
them.

Although they may not be aware of their prejudices,
these so-called care-givers subtly or blatantly look down
on you and make you feel that you're cantankerous or
childlike, a complainer or a hypochondriac. They may
shout when they speak to you (assuming that you're
deaf) or suggest that since you're eighty-seven, you
should *expect* to feel dizzy when you get up in the
morning or that it's normal to be exhausted at four
o'clock every afternoon. If you're not sure of their attitude, but you end up feeling bad or stupid when they
leave your bedside or when you leave their office, that's

a good indicator that their attitude toward you is less than desirable.

The same goes for doctors who treat older women in a negative or offhand manner. There's no reason that older women should be treated as ''old biddies'' or ''hysterical women'' whose complaints are not taken seriously.

Even when they're very sick, women (and men) must learn to assert themselves on their own behalf in these situations. ''Sharon Sommers'' had always been healthy, with the exception of pneumonia, which she'd had in her early fifties. One evening after dinner, however, she found herself doubled over in pain. Her husband Bill drove her to the nearest emergency room.

''I spent two and a half hours in the emergency room,'' she said, ''and all they did was take my temperature. They didn't give me blood tests or anything. The doctor asked me how was my marriage and whether I'd been upset by anything lately. He treated me like a hysterical woman and told me to go home and take a hot shower. He sounded quite official—like he knew what he was talking about. The next night after dinner, I was in tremendous pain again. I got into the shower and as I was standing there, I thought, 'If they don't take care of me, I'm going to die.' Bill took me back to the emergency room, and we insisted that I be given some kind of tests. The doctor acted perturbed, as if I was being a naughty child, but then another doctor came in and talked with me. He did some tests and when he came back in, he said, 'I apologize. You have a gall-bladder problem. It's a pancreatic infection. I'm afraid you weren't treated very well last night.'

''I was in such pain that I could barely fight. I don't know what would have happened if Bill hadn't been there to back me up. When you're sick, it's hard. But now I know something. I know to say, 'Before you tell me it's my age, or I'm hysterical—obviously because

302 THE SAFE MEDICINE BOOK

I'm a woman—I want a better answer! I've got to know why I feel this way!' ''

The Importance of a Doctor You Trust
If you visit a doctor who trivializes your complaints, who rushes you in and out, who doesn't listen to your symptoms or speak to you as an intelligent person interested in making good, well-informed decisions, find a different doctor. Don't let the doctor tell you your symptoms are all in your mind when you are feeling pains you never had before, seeing yellow circles in front of your eyes, or noticing a new bend or angle in your back.

Dr. Butler advises that if you have a doctor who clearly doesn't care about your feelings or your questions, *change doctors*. Even though you may be perfectly healthy now, would you want to be cared for during a serious illness by someone with such negative attitudes? Would you trust him or her to make decisions on your behalf if you were unconscious?

Some doctors are better than others at helping you feel comfortable and responsible. Trust your own instincts. Ask yourself if your doctor makes sense to you. Is your doctor willing to involve you and educate you? Does your doctor listen to you? Do you feel that she cares about what happens to you?

If you're over sixty-five, it may be advisable for you to go to a geriatrician rather than to a doctor who doesn't seem aware of differences between normal aging and pathological disease. Geriatricians are doctors who have studied the physiology and pathology of old age. They have chosen to specialize in understanding elderly patients and to spend their professional lives with them. This choice usually indicates a special regard for matters that concern you. Aware of social and nutritional problems, for instance, geriatricians often work in close contact with nutritionists and social workers. They realize that certain problems like transportation or physical mobility can make a difference in your ability to carry out your treatment plan. And they know that the way you deal with the death of a spouse is as critical to your health as the way you would deal with a new disease. Probably one of the most important features of geriatric medicine is that, by its very orientation, it values the dignity and independence of your life. "I heard the geriatrician defined as the only doctor who's willing to listen to the patient and stop a medication," says Dr. Michael Freedman. "But I think that one of the most important things that geriatrics has done is to recognize that the elderly deserve to live a quality life."

While a doctor who hasn't been trained in geriatrics might never stop to think that an eighty-year-old has an active sex life she wants to maintain, a geriatrician would know to ask before writing a prescription that could interfere with her libido. And similarly, a doctor who doesn't know that an eighty-four-year-old plans to celebrate his hundred-and-fourth birthday, just like his grandfather did, might not bother to take emergency measures if they were needed.

"Four years ago when I wanted to have surgery on my arm so I could move it better, I saw this doctor who had the viewpoint that I didn't have much longer to live anyway, so why should he bother?" says eighty-two-year-old "Florrie Rothman," who found a different surgeon to operate on her. "I really resented that he wouldn't do for me what he would do for someone younger. Who was he to decide I didn't have that much longer to live? I may outlive him! I may have another twenty-five years, for all he knows.

"I have never felt old. Sometimes I get a little shocked when I'm walking by a store window and I realize that the little gray-haired lady reflected in the window is me. But then I think, 'Well, not that many people are walking as briskly as I am, either.' The last few times I went for walks with my daughters-in-law, I had to slow down for them."

Dr. Freedman also tells a story of a seventy-three-year-old man who came into the hospital with acute leukemia a number of years ago. He wanted to be treated for the leukemia, but an internist he saw said it just wasn't worth his time, presumably because he was just an old man who was going to die soon anyway. Dr. Freedman stumbled onto the case and insisted on having the patient attended to. "We treated him," says Dr. Freedman, "and he went into complete remission! Over the years, he's sent me cards and kept me up-to-date on what he's doing. Last month I got a letter from him that had a Florida postmark. He said, 'I just wanted to let you know that we're living in Florida now because my wife is sick. I want to thank you again for keeping me alive fifteen years ago, because if I were not here, my wife wouldn't have anyone to take care of her and she would have to be put in a nursing home.' "

Geriatricians are in short supply throughout the United States, but there are internists and family practitioners who also have a commitment to your health and well-being. Although they may not have been trained specifically in geriatrics, they may be very well informed about aging and disease.

"Doctors don't need to know about the elderly so much as they need to be attentive to change," says pharmaceutical consultant Randall Wright. "They need to recognize if their patient is walking differently than he did the last time. What you look for is changes and what causes the changes. Then you look for what will make a difference when those changes are harmful."

If you live in a small town and have no alternative to a doctor who tells you that you should expect what you're experiencing because you're old, educate him. Tell your physician that you understand that a lot of doctors don't know much about older people or the process of aging, but clearly it's time he became educated. Don't let your doctor get away with "ageist" attitudes.

As gerontologist Myrna Lewis said, "Patients are going to have to lead their doctors by the hand into the twenty-first century.''

Dealing with More than One Doctor

When you deal with just one doctor, it should be relatively easy to ask questions and get answers. But if you go to a heart specialist, a dentist, a podiatrist, a psychiatrist, an internist, and a gynecologist, will you remember to tell each of them what the others have prescribed? Will you tell them to talk to one another?

When there is no one person in charge of your program and committed to following through on your case, big mistakes can be made. Something as simple as being seen by a second doctor in a group practice can lead to a lack of important doctor-patient communication.

Fortunately, the grave lack of communication in Alvin Ahern's case didn't take his life, but it well might have.

When he was eighty, Dr. Ahern, former dean of the New York Theological Seminary in New York City, was sent by his internist to the Charlotte Hungerford Hospital in Torrington, Connecticut, to take a stress test. ''After a short period of walking on the treadmill, the test was interrupted,'' he says, ''leaving me with the impression that they'd found no problem.

''My doctor's associate, who was monitoring the test, said, 'Your doctor will talk to you about this.' My doctor's colleague didn't say anything else one way or another. A day or so after we got home, we called in and asked about the test results and the nurse said, 'The doctor will get back to you when he gets the report.'

''Three weeks later, during my normal checkup with my doctor, I asked him about the results of the stress test. He said, 'Let me see, I'll go find out.' That was eleven A.M. He came back and said, 'I'm going to refer you to a cardiologist today. You have a heart condition that's life-threatening.' It appeared to me that his associate had never told him how bad the test was! By two P.M., I was in a Dr. O'Reilly's office. He gave me a complete exam and recommended me to a heart surgeon named Dr. Low. They gave me an angiogram; then they all conferred and strongly advised cardiovascular surgery. Bypass. I asked the cardiologist if the test results indicated surgery. He said, 'They *mandate* it.' ''

"He had a triple bypass," Dr. Ahern's wife, Helen, asserts. "During those three weeks when we thought the results of the stress test had been positive, he had been out splitting wood. He was using the wedge. He could have died over those chunks of wood. We didn't worry about it at the time, though. It was the comfort of ignorance!"

To make sure that this kind of potential accident doesn't happen to you, find one central person who will coordinate your health care. This person should receive copies of your test results, diagnosis, and treatment plans, including medications prescribed, from other physicians. With the many forms of medical care that are emerging today, from group practice to HMOs, it can be difficult to find such a coordinator. Often, however, your internist or family practitioner will be glad to receive these reports from other doctors. It also may be that he'll ask his physician's assistant or nurse to do the job.

Today, with the many forms of medical care emerging, from group practice to HMOs and other health-care conglomerates, it's particularly difficult, but important, for you to make sure that one central person is aware of all aspects of your medical history, your health, your tests, and your medications. This person may end up being a physician, a physician's assistant, or a nurse, but this person should coordinate communication on critical issues involving your health and medical welfare. You will need to ask specialists or other health-care professionals to send your coordinator copies of test results, diagnosis, and treatment plans, including medications, so that your health care is co-ordinated and doesn't work against itself.

If you are going to a clinic or an HMO, Dr. Meier recommends that you ask about the focus and coordination of your program. ''Express what you think to the physician you see,'' she says. ''Tell her, 'I know I can get good health care here, but there's always the risk of fragmented and disjointed care, and I'd like you to oversee my program.' It's all about being an informed and enlightened consumer.''

Remember, when you see a doctor, even in emergency situations:

- You have the right to be respected.
- You have the right to ask questions and get straight-forward answers to those questions.
- You have the right to know your diagnosis.
- You have the right to know the risks involved in your treatment and choose accordingly.
- You are purchasing the service of the doctor; you have the right to know his opinion, to explore your alternatives—to know what might be done to you and why. You have the right to select or refuse treatments that affect your health and well-being.
- You have the right to a second opinion.
- You have the right to change doctors.
- You have the right—and the duty—to stand up for yourself and assert your prerogative to get the best health care possible.

PREPARING FOR YOUR VISIT TO THE DOCTOR

When you make an appointment to see the doctor, prepare in advance for your visit. Start a few days ahead of time. If you have been feeling ill, get a notebook and write down a list of the ways you have been feeling. If you don't make notes, it's easy to forget whether you have the sharp pains upon awakening or immediately following a meal. You may forget that you also have headaches during a certain time of day. That's why a list is helpful. It will give you a reference for answering the doctor's questions as well as covering all your own.

Write down the following:

* Your complaints, if you have any. What has been bothering you?
* Your symptoms. If it's a pain, is it sharp? Is it dull?
* How long have you been feeling this way?
* When did it start? What happened when you first noticed it?
* If and when it has ever happened before.
* If so, how it was treated.
* Your medical history, your chronic or underlying disorders, such as high blood pressure, glaucoma, diabetes, or heart disease. (If you are going to a clinic, an HMO, or a new doctor, take along your medical records.)
* All the drugs you use, meaning all prescription drugs and over-the-counter drugs including vitamins, aspirin, eye drops, laxatives, and antacids.
* The amount of alcohol you drink on a daily basis.
* Any allergies you have to foods or medications.
* Any bad side effects or adverse reactions you've had to previous medications.
* Any questions you have about your conditions.

Prepare this list over several days' time, since some questions only pop into your mind every now and then and can pop out during a short interview, when you might be feeling stressed or distracted.

On the day of your doctor's appointment, remember to take along your list and ask the doctor your questions. Don't worry that you will be taking up too much of your doctor's time.

Dr. Butler and other geriatricians recommend that

when you go to see your doctor, you should ask for "the brown-bag" medicine check. Take along a brown bag or plastic bag full of all your pills, ointments, eye drops,
vitamins, and nonprescription medicines. Let the doctor look at them and ask you questions about them. He or his assistant or nurse can check the expiration dates and find out what you're taking that possibly conflicts. Don't forget to include everything from aspirin to Alka-Seltzer to Tums.

Even when you've been seeing the same doctor for quite some time, you can ask him for a brown-bag check. It may be that you have some old medications or some duplications in your medicine cabinet. It may be that you're still taking a medicine that you don't need anymore. Ask your doctor if there's any medicine you can stop taking. For instance, if you've changed your diet and your blood pressure is down, do you still need your high blood pressure medicine?

Always ask your doctor if there's any alternative to medication. The view that all ailments and diseases can best be treated with some kind of medicine simply isn't true. Because people believe that they "need" a prescription, doctors often feel pressured into writing one— and people end up taking drugs they don't need. Drugs, as we've learned, involve health risks, especially for older people. Often we can learn to cope in new ways with certain discomforts or conditions we assumed needed medication. This can make us feel stronger, healthier, and more self-reliant. Even if you've been taking a tranquilizer or a sleeping pill for a number of years, you might try to work with your doctor on getting off the medication. It may well be that you don't need it anymore.

"Most doctors love it when a patient comes in and asks, 'Is there something else I can do besides medications?' " says Dr. Michael Freedman, director of the Division of Geriatrics at New York University Medical

Center. "It's a refreshing change from the patients who come in and say, 'Aren't you going to give me a pill?' "

Talking About the Prescription

If your doctor tells you that a particular medication is necessary, and if you're convinced that the benefits of this particular drug outweigh its risks, then you are ready to take charge of it. Remember all that you've learned about handling your medications. Make sure that the prescription is legible and that you know its purpose and what to expect from it. Find out what foods and beverages you should avoid, and whether to take the medicine with, before, or after meals. (Refer to the checklist at the back of the book.) Also make sure you know how often to take the medicine and for how long. If your doctor clearly doesn't know about the medicine's interactive effects with foods, ask him if he can recommend a good nutritionist who could help you with your diet. Before you leave his office, find out when you're supposed to see him or contact him again.

Remember, some drugs the doctor prescribes for serious illnesses are lethal. Some cancer drugs, for instance, are pure poison. The risks with some others aren't so serious, but they have severe side effects. Don't forget that it's your decision whether or not you want to take them.

For some medications or injections, you'll be asked to sign a consent form. Don't sign the form unless you understand very clearly what risks are involved and unless you're willing to take those risks. You don't have to sign the forms while you're at the doctor's office. Go home and think it over if you want to. Get a second opinion if you want to.

After You're at Home

Remember, after you get home from the doctor's office and the pharmacy, be aware of how you are feeling. Once you start taking a medication, pay attention to any stomach cramps, dizziness, or other discomforts you may experience. Remember that yours is a unique system.

Remember also:

- Don't mix medications unless your physician or pharmacist has told you that you may do so.
- Don't drive a car, operate heavy machinery, or attempt any complicated task that involves heavy objects unless you're sure how that medication affects you.

If you detect any unusual changes after taking a medicine, call your doctor, dentist, nurse, or pharmacist and tell them what is happening to you. If you get sick, or sicker, your medication be the prime suspect.

CHAPTER 13

Setting Up for Safety—Dos and Don'ts of Managing Your Medications

> If you want to be cured of I don't know what, take this herb of I don't know what name, apply it I don't know where, and you will be cured I don't know when.
>
> —MEDIEVAL JOCOSITY,
> SOURCE UNKNOWN

> There is a common argument that is both false and fatal. "So-and-so," one hears, "has been cured by such-and-such a treatment, and I have his disease; ergo, I must try his remedy." How many people die by reasoning thus! What they overlook is that the diseases which affect us are as different as the features of our faces.
>
> —VOLTAIRE; LETTER TO
> BARON DE BRETUIL,
> DECEMBER 1723.

No matter how smart you are, it's easy to be dumb about using your medications. Recently, for instance, a very smart friend of mine called me up and left a message on my telephone answering machine. "Look to see if you have anything for conjunctivitis," she said. "If you do, bring it over when you come for dinner."

When I listened to the message, I thought how easy it might be to "help out" in a case like this. If I'd previously had an eye infection (and I didn't know better), I might have rummaged through my medicine cabinet and come up with what was left of a tube of medication my doctor had prescribed for me. I imagined some of the horrible possibilities:

- It might have helped me, but it might contain an ingredient my friend is allergic to. She puts it in her eye and it swells up instantly. As a result, she loses partial sight, or, worse, goes blind.
- It might be that I had a different eye infection and that I had touched the tube to my eyelid putting it in. I imagined her touching it to her eyelid, getting bacteria from it, and getting a horrible eye infection as a result.
- It might be that she doesn't have conjunctivitis at all, but a red and itchy eye that's indicative of something else. My medication could damage her sight, make her sick, or let her temporarily ignore a serious symptom.
- She may have exactly what I had but my medicine may not be good anymore and her infection may get worse while she's using a tube of medicine that should have been thrown away long ago.

The incident made me think of an interview I'd had with Esther Sobering, administrator of the Home Health Services for Riley County, Kansas, when she said, "I don't think the elderly are any dumber or any smarter than young people when it comes to their medications. Correcting the problems is just a matter of taking medicines as prescribed by the physician and *not* taking medicine *not* prescribed by the physician."

Studies show that misuse of their medications is a significant problem with all age groups, but it's an even greater problem for people over sixty-five. A variety of studies indicates that *more than half of people sixty-five and over do not take their medications as prescribed*. Patients who report on the intake of their medications tend to be optimistic in terms of their compliance. Records of pills actually taken compared to what the patient *says* indicate that patients are mistaken in favor of their consistency by 20 or 30 percent.

In addition to the serious problems we've described (multiple drugs, interactions of drugs and disease, failure to adjust the prescription to the aging body, overdoses, mixing OTCs with prescription drugs, side effects or adverse drug reactions or failure to get or understand instructions), pharmacists, nurses, and social workers report that the main problems with patients complying with their drug regimens seem to be:

- *Not filling the prescription in the first place.* Some 10 percent of the elderly never get the prescription filled. This may be because the medicine is expensive and they can't afford it, or because they decide on their own that they don't need the medicine.

- *Not taking the full dose.* When people feel bad, they take the medicine because they want to feel better. If they feel better, they don't see the need to take the medicine anymore. This is okay some of the time, but it's not okay especially when it comes to certain antibiotics or to blood pressure medicine. (If you're on tetracycline, for instance, stopping before the full regime is completed makes the treatment ineffective.)

- *Not being able to get the top off the bottle.* Sometimes people with arthritic fingers get home and can't get the cap off a "childproof" container. The frustration sometimes makes the struggle too much to cope with. Even if someone else takes the cap off and then puts it back on, the patient is confronted with the same problem the next time he wants to use the medicine.

- *Forgetting to take medicine.* Studies show that people sometimes simply forget to take their medicines. These errors are potentially quite serious.

- *Taking too much medicine.* Sometimes people duplicate one prescription. They'll go to several physicians who prescribe similar drugs and not tell them what else they're taking. This is a chief factor in overdose problems.

- *Assuming that if one is good, two is better.* Another serious cause of overdosing is the belief that if one pill has made you feel better, then two pills will make you get better faster. Sometimes people also take two pills at once to compensate for having missed a dose they were supposed to take four hours ago. They think that since they forgot that one, taking two now will make up for it. This can make you very sick.

- *Swapping medicines, sharing prescriptions, or taking medicines they shouldn't.* One of the reasons people swap or share medicines is that they think it will save them money. If Mrs. Jones has the same thing Mrs. Smith had last year, and Mrs. Smith has some medicine left, she'll give some of it to Mrs. Jones. They seem to have the same symptoms, and this will save Mrs. Jones some money. This isn't really helpful or cost-effective in the long run. Mrs. Smith's prescription may be old and ineffective, or even if it's the same substance, it may be five milligrams instead of two milligrams. It may be compounded with another drug that would be harmful to Mrs. Smith.

- *Inability to distinguish one medicine from another.* Sometimes two entirely different pills are the same color and shape. If the medication containers are not clearly marked, it's easy to confuse them. Sometimes, if you have a vision problem it's difficult to read the medicine labels and keep track of what pill you've taken and what pill you haven't taken. Another visual problem can occur if patients who can't distinguish well between colors are instructed to take "the blue pill" at such and such a time and the "green pill" at another time. Some older eyes lose their ability to distinguish between colors, and when it comes to mistakes between pills, it can be a disaster.

* *Using expired drugs.* People who have hoarded their medications often pull them out to use again for new symptoms. If they used something five years ago for a bad headache, they think it will help again this time. Sometimes this medication has deteriorated. After the expiration date, it can change chemically and become more potent or less potent or have no effect at all. Sometimes the spoiled medication, which would not have been knowingly prescribed because of another, more recent condition, will make the patient sick or will duplicate or interact adversely with other medications.

* *Getting confused about when to take your medicine.* Particularly if you're taking several medications, it's easy to get into trouble from not following the proper schedule. For example, if you're supposed to take one capsule four times daily and two tablets twice daily, it's easy to get confused and start taking one tablet four times a day and two capsules two times day. Unless you set up a predictable routine, taking too many or too few pills can become the rule, not the exception.

It Happens to Everyone

Don't worry that you're getting senile if you've mismanaged your medications. Even when you're surrounded by medical people, it can still happen to you.

When Sylvia McBurnie's stepfather was sick, for instance, Sylvia noticed a number of medications on the table beside his bed. She began to examine them and found that there were several different prescriptions for the same drug.

"I first looked at the names of the drugs and realized there were several of the same drug with different names," said the former associate director of Nursing for Geriatrics at Mount Sinai Hospital. "There were different colors and shapes, depending on the company that manufactured them. Some were brand names and some were generic. He didn't realize that the medicines were the same thing.

"He was really overmedicated. Here he was, the husband of a nurse and the stepfather of a nurse, and no one had noticed!

"Next I started looking at expiration dates on the bottles and I discovered that quite a few of them were long past their expiration dates!"

Sylvia McBurnie ended up throwing out more than three-fourths of her stepfather's medications. She talked with his doctor about what he really needed and what he could do without. Her experience startled her and made her realize that people know very little about their medications.

A Follow-Up on Compliance

A lot of research has been done on how patients misuse their medicines, but very little has been done to improve the situation. Recently, however, an innovative project aimed at providing solutions to the follow-up and monitoring of patients on blood pressure medications has gotten under way at Boston University School of Medicine. It may serve as a model for helping older people manage their treatment plans for a variety of medical conditions and reduce problems that result from medication misuse.

In the project, run by the Medical Information Systems Unit at Boston University School of Medicine, fifty people in the greater Boston area are being contacted at least once a week to find out whether they're taking their medications and how they're reacting to them. They're also asked about other things that could affect their condition, such as diet and exercise. What makes this project particularly interesting is that a

318 THE SAFE MEDICINE BOOK

telephone-linked computer system plays the role of visiting nurse.

Dr. Robert Friedman, chief of the Medical Information Systems Unit and director of the Telephone-Linked Computer (TLC) system, explains that patients trained for the project are encouraged to call the computer once a week between doctor visits. If they don't call, the computer calls them.

Over the telephone, the patient, along with all the details of his individual medical history, is identified by a word code. The patient, who is supposed to take his blood pressure daily, reports it. The computer knows the target blood pressure, the medications the patient should be taking, the schedule for taking them, and the potential side effects. It knows whether or not the patient has taken this medication in the past.

By means of a speech-synthesis device that converts signals into sounds, the computer has a human-sounding voice tailored to the needs of the listener—increasing high-frequency tones, slowing the voice down, or increasing the volume if needed. During each interchange, the computer asks the most important questions and makes a response to the answers it gets. It decides what to say based on very specific and targeted goals.

For instance, when the patient tells the computer what his blood pressure is, it may respond to the patient, ''I want you to know that your blood pressure is much better than last time.'' If the patient is taking his medication as scheduled, the computer response reinforces the behavior with positive comments. If the blood pressure isn't good, the computer will say something like, ''Your blood pressure is a little high today, and you're telling me you're not taking your medicines half of the time. If you take it regularly, it will probably improve. Why don't you call me back in two days and tell me how it is?''

The TLC system automatically prints out a ''lab report'' containing the blood pressure results and other information reported by the patient and sends it to the doctor. If the patient has an emergency situation, the computer calls the physician's office and says, "I just talked to your patient and he doesn't know what he's doing. His blood pressure is very high."

Dr. Friedman expects that eventually the monitoring system will be used in elderly housing and home-care settings to allow older people to maintain independent living and still be monitored. Currently, along with the New England Research Institute, he is planning an expanded program involving some six hundred people over the age of sixty in seven communities surrounding Boston.

"Noncompliance with the taking of medications may be more common with the elderly simply because they take more medications," says Dr. Friedman. "But the situation is critical for older people because their margin of safety is much less than with younger people. Doctors know about it, but they don't have very good ways of dealing with it.

"The interest of the physicians in finding out whether their patients are taking medications as prescribed varies widely. Relatively few do it systematically.

"We have high hopes for this system," says Dr. Friedman. "It's very inexpensive. We figure that to monitor one person once a week for a year, it costs about twenty or thirty dollars total. Just to send one person to a patient's home once costs more than that. Even if you could hire a person to make calls to patients, it would be more than that. Besides, the computer can call thousands of people and adjust the timing of the calls to fit their schedules. It can call at night, early in the morning, anytime."

SAVE YOUR MONEY AND YOUR HEALTH

In the long run, you'll save money in doctor's bills and in hospital bills if you take your medications properly. You may not have a computer checking up on you every week, but you can provide your own monitoring system. Rules and regulations that will help you avoid problems include the following maxims:

- Fill your prescription. If you don't fill it, tell your doctor you didn't fill it and why.
- Know the names of your medications and why you are taking them.
- In general, keep your pills in their original container. It contains all the information you need on the label. If you need to report back to your pharmacist for a refill, for instance, he'll ask you for the prescription number. If you're ever feeling groggy or distracted, you can still read the label before taking any pill. (The one exception to this rule comes if you are using a pill dispenser or putting your pills into a daily compartment. If you put your pills into a weekly or monthly pill dispenser, make sure that the medications are *clearly* labeled and save the original container.)
- Make sure you can read the label on your prescription. The complete label should include your name, your doctor's name, the name of the drug, the prescription number, instructions for use, the date the prescription was filled, and the expiration date.
- Additionally, ask your pharmacist to mark on your label what each medication is for. For instance, ask him to write *heart pill* beside *digoxin* or *blood pressure* by *Corgard*.
- If you have difficulty reading fine print, ask your nurse or pharmacist to write the label and exact directions for how and when to take your medicine in *big* letters.

- Make sure you can open your pill container before you leave the pharmacy.
- Ask your pharmacist for written information on the medication as well as what he's told you verbally.
- Don't duplicate your dosages. Don't take two pills if you forgot to take one four hours ago.
- Ask your pharmacist or doctor what to do if you forgot to take your medicine.
- Don't share your medicines.
- Don't take anyone else's medicines. Don't borrow and don't loan them, even for the same condition.
- Two is *not* better than one.
- Don't decide for yourself what medicines you should take and then take old ones. Talk to your doctor first.
- Keep a drug diary of your medications, noting the date the drug was prescribed, how much you were given and how often, and how long you took it. Note any side effects, allergic reactions, or adverse reactions.
- Don't collect or save your medications. Take them for as long as the doctor tells you and then toss them out.
- Toss out any medications that have an expired date.
- If you are *sure* that you will be using these medications again and want to save them, check with your pharmacist. Perhaps he will tell you where to save them or he will hold them for you.
- Call your doctor or your pharmacist if you experience side effects or adverse reactions.
- Write down exactly what foods or beverages you should or should not mix with your medicine.
- Find out whether the medication will deplete any vitamins or minerals from your system, and whether you should take a food supplement to make up for the loss.
- Ask whether you need to take this food on an empty stomach or before, after, or between meals. Write down your instructions.

- Don't drink milk or eat other dairy products such as cheese or yogurt if you are taking tetracycline. This antibiotic also shouldn't be mixed with antacids, calcium, or iron preparations.
- Always take your medicine with a full glass of water. Water helps it dissolve properly. Don't take your medicine with a cola, a soda, or orange juice. The acid in these drinks may make the medicine dissolve too quickly for it to be properly absorbed.
- If you're on any MAO inhibitor for depression, totally avoid beer, wine, cheese, salami, pickles, and the other foods mentioned in Chapter 8, because the mixture can be fatal.
- Don't drink alcohol if you are taking antihistamines, tranquilizers, barbiturates, or antidepressants. These combinations can be dangerous.

As I've said before, and it bears repeating, your pharmacist is a valuable source of information. A pharmacist you know and trust is also in the position to spot any problems in terms of dosages or adverse drug interactions *before* they happen. As Dr. James W. Cooper at the University of Georgia's College of Pharmacy says, "The *role* of the pharmacist is to intervene on behalf of his patients. That's what we're there for!"

Your pharmacist can also help you by explaining *how* to take the drug and *when* to take it. He can tell you what to do if you miss one dose or several doses. If you have a pill you're only supposed to take once a day, your pharmacist can tell you whether it would be better for you to take it in the morning or the evening—and *why* it would be better. Your pharmacist can also answer questions about side effects and help you figure out a schedule for taking your medicines.

Nurses, too, are wonderful sources for setting up a good system that will help you remember to take your medications. Usually home nurses go through the medicine cabinets of their patients to check expiration dates and duplications. They are excellent at helping you figure out what works best for you.

Organizing for Safety

A daily regimen is very important for proper use of medications. If you're taking more than one medicine, it's particularly imperative that you be on a coordinated and controlled schedule. Some tips I've gotten from pharmacists and nurses on setting up and following a safe and individualized medicine regimen are the following:

- Read the label on your prescription *each time* you take your medicine. Prescription vials do look alike, and getting them mixed up can mean serious trouble for you.
- Take the exact dose that's been prescribed for you. If you're taking a liquid medication, measure it exactly. Use measuring spoons intended for cooking.
- Work out a plan that is as simple as possible for taking your medicines.
- Try to fit the pill-taking schedule in with your daily routine. If, for instance, you spray your plants every morning, that might be a good time to take your daily pill. A system that helps you remember by association is usually a system that works (for example, you might remember to take your medicine when you feed your cat every morning and evening or when you brush your hair).
- If you're taking more than one medication, set up your "swallow chart" on a large schedule or calendar and make a check mark each time you take the medicine you're supposed to take. No matter how good your memory is, this is a very helpful method. It's easy to forget whether or not you took medicine at noon, but when you're using a chart, you can confirm your suspicions.
- Another thing that can help is a pillbox that has di-

visions for each day of the week. Unfortunately, pills you have to take on a long-term basis aren't divided into ''dose'' packs as birth control pills are. A weekly pillbox divided into seven rows of three or four compartments, however, can be almost as helpful. Pills for each ''pill-taking time'' can be sorted out at the beginning of the week and put into their proper compartment. Smaller devices may have certain compartments marked for 8:00 A.M., 12:00 noon, and 6:00 P.M. When it's time to take your pills, you simply go to your pillbox and take out the pills for that occasion. This is also an easy way to see whether or not you remembered to take your pills at the last designated time.

- An egg carton can be an effective organizer for pills. You can mark days of the week or certain times of the day and set it up each morning. Obviously, if you have trouble doing this for yourself, a visiting nurse or a friend or relative could also set it up for you.

- If you take pills three times a day, you may want to have one pillbox with compartments or even three separate pillboxes—each distinct from the others—that you set out each morning. It simplifies the routine and insures that you have your pills with you no matter where you are.

- Some medicines must not be exposed to light or to air because they will decompose. If you are planning to set out your medications in a pillbox or egg carton, check with your pharmacist to make sure that they won't deteriorate.

- If you have trouble with your sight and have a problem distinguishing between pills, ask your pharmacist or nurse to help you alter the containers so that they're recognizable. For instance, the pill that you're supposed to take three times a day is in the big bottle. The pill that you're supposed to take before you go to bed at night is in the small round bottle with the rough cap. Ways of distinguishing between bottles and pills can include putting rubber bands around a certain bottle or fastening rough sandpaper around the sides of another.

- If you have trouble remembering when to take a certain medication, set an alarm or ask a friend or family member to call and remind you to take your medicine.

- Nurses will also take the time to teach you how to take your medicine the proper way. If you have questions, ask. They have the medical knowledge and the practical experience in how to set things up so that they work for you.

- Currently new innovations are being explored that will help with remembering when to take your medications. Recently, for instance, a pill bottle has been developed that has a small computer chip in the lid. When it's time to take your pill, the lid beeps—just like an alarm clock—to wake you up and remind you to take your medicine.

Learning New Tricks

More and more older people are going to be managing their own health care within their homes. Currently, a large number of people over eighty-five who could be cared for in nursing homes are opting to stay at home for financial or emotional reasons. Also, people are being sent home from their hospital stays more quickly. While it used to be that people would spend ten days in the hospital, now they'll spend three and have home-health nurses stop in to visit them for a week afterward. At home, these people will usually not have the kind of medical supervision they would have in a hospital or nursing home—and sometimes managing their medications is a very challenging task. This is particularly so when they have special disabilities.

"Just because you're old doesn't make you incapacitated," says Esther Sobering. "Most people can be taught to live independently with a little advice and a change of habit. For instance, a person whose arm shakes can learn to lean against a wall and support her arm against a cupboard to get the eye drops in correctly.''

According to Ms. Sobering, a lot of people are sent home from the hospital with tube feedings that need to be managed. ''Sometimes we don't think of this as medication, but it is because it's regulated. People have to be taught how to manage their own tube feedings, how to change the tube and check the solution.

''More and more [health care] is being done in the home. The family is taught what to do for the patient, and the home-health nurses provide support and supervision. The biggest change is that health care is no longer being seen as such a secretive thing. People can learn about it. If one person can learn it, so can another.''

One of the main functions of home-health nurses is to teach patients how to take care of themselves. These lessons can be invaluable for helping older people remain independent and in control of their own experiences.

A New Jersey home-health nurse told me about working out a home health-care plan with a woman in her early eighties who was blind. ''Mrs. White'' had been a businesswoman most of her life and now lived in a high-rise apartment. She'd recently had cataract surgery, was mildly diabetic, and was taking heart medicine. She could see light and dark but nothing more. Nevertheless, she was a very independent person and had a real desire to function effectively on her own.

''Right after her cataract surgery, when she came home, she needed some help,'' said her nurse. ''We went in every four hours. She had to take pills for her heart plus eye drops. Also, she was on a diabetic diet and she had Meals On Wheels brought in.

''In the hospital they'd added a new heart medicine

to her regimen that was strange to her, plus she had two eye drops for the operated eye and one for the other eye. We had to keep all that straight. At first we did it, but we figured that after the nurses stopped going in four times a day, she had to know how to do it for herself.

"That's when we set up different containers for her. We gave her a large container with a rubber band around it for her old heart medicine, which she took once a day. Then we got a small, properly labeled container for the new medicine. She could tell quite easily which container was which.

"We asked her if she had any friends on her floor, and she said yes, she had one. Mrs. White invited her over, and we talked with her and asked her to come in and help with the eye drops. She was glad to help. Mrs. White would lean her head back and her friend would just drop in the drops. It took about a minute.

"Usually we teach people to put all their medications in one place all the time," said the nurse. "That way they don't misplace or forget them. But we put Mrs. White's eye drops in one place and her pills in another place that was close by, so she wouldn't confuse them.

"Most doctors don't think about this kind of thing when they give prescriptions, but they should."

Where to Keep Your Medicines

Most of us store our medicines in the bathroom because the medicine cabinet is located there. Unfortunately, this is not a good idea. Pharmacists say that the best place to keep most prescription drugs is someplace that is dry and cool. Good places are in a hall cupboard or linen closet. Sometimes there's a shelf in a closet or a special spot in the top dresser drawer. The bathroom is moist and warm and thus not a good spot. Temperature and humidity can make a big difference in the potency and effectiveness of medicines. Other rules of thumb include the following:

- Some medicines need to be refrigerated. Look at the label to see what it says, or ask your pharmacist where and how the medicine should be stored. Many liquid medicines must be refrigerated or they will lose their potency.
- Some drugs have to be sealed in dark containers. They should not be exposed to light or air because light and air help decompose them.
- Patients who are diabetic and test their urine with pills have to be careful about where and how they store those pills. Clini-Tek or Acitest pills have to be tightly sealed in dark bottles. Patients need to be aware if the pills change color. Sometimes you can't see the change.
- Don't keep medicines on the table beside your bed. It's easy to imagine how you might reach for a medicine and get the wrong bottle. It's also easy to imagine that if you have sleeping pills, tranquilizers, or sedatives by your bed, you may forget you already took a pill and take a second. Don't take that chance.
- Don't take medicine in the dark. Turn on the light and read the label.
- Keep the medicine out of reach of your grandchildren, neighbors, or any small children. According to the U.S. Consumer Product Safety Commission, some 36 percent of all prescription drug poisoning by young children involves a grandparent's medication.
- Teach children to respect drugs, and avoid taking your medicine in front of very small children if you can. Don't refer to it as "candy." If they see you taking it, explain its purpose and make sure to put it away immediately after using it.

Day-to-Day Precautions
When I visited the senior center in Saint Marys, Kansas, I asked several people what sort of day-to-day pre-

cautions they took in terms of their health and medication.

"Everybody knows everybody else here," said Henry Quigley. "That's one of the reasons my wife and I moved back here from Topeka. It's good for our health! It's a good feeling to know that you're known."

Rita Meyer, who's sixty-nine years old, pulled a small blue book out of her purse. "This is what I carry," she said. "It's got all the details anybody would need to know, just in case."

The small blue book Rita Meyer was carrying was "Passport to Good Health" and is published by the National Institute on Drug Abuse. Inside, Rita had written her name, address, and telephone number and her doctor's name and telephone number.

In the front of the book, she listed the prescription medications she was on and wrote down what they looked like and what they were for. Her list said, as follows:

Pronestyl, 375 mg, one cap four times daily for high blood pressure (orange and white, oblong)

Aldomet, 250 mg, one tab three times daily for pressure (yellow pill, round)

K-Lor, 20 mg, potassium a day

Terramycin, 250 mg, one four times daily for sinus infection

Triavil, 2/25 A.M. and P.M., for nerves (triangle-shaped)

Kinesed, one tab four times daily as needed for indigestion (orange, oblong).

There were also spaces in the book for "Allergies or Reactions" and "Directions" and "Cautions." Although she's surrounded by friends and neighbors who know her and know her doctor, Mrs. Meyer's precautions make a lot of sense. She could be on any kind of medication—and her friends might not know it. Also, if she ever required emergency treatment when she was away from home, her "passport" could be a lifesaver.

Dr. Michael Freedman of New York University Medical Center, in reviewing this list, pointed out that even though Mrs. Meyer keeps accurate records of what she's taking, this combination of medications could cause many problems. For example, Aldomet, an antihypertensive, may cause depression, he says. It is conceivable that Triavil was prescribed to Mrs. Meyer to treat her depression. However, Triavil can cause cardiac arrhythmias. Therefore, it is also conceivable that Pronestyl was prescribed to treat the cardiac arrhythmias. So it is quite possible that Mrs. Meyer, rather than experiencing depression and arrhythmias, could have been prescribed an alternative antihypertensive and knocked two medications off her list in the process.

Besides being on as few drugs as possible and keeping a record of your medicines, what other day-to-day precautions are important for you to take in case you faint or pass out when you're in the middle of JC Penney's, if you're just walking down the street by yourself, or if you faint after having won the jackpot on a one-armed bandit in Las Vegas?

"At our senior centers we have a lot of emergencies," said Marlene Asherman, a social worker in New York City. "People faint or have a heart attack or are clearly in critical situations. The first questions are whom do we call? What are they taking? What are their special problems?"

If you have any allergies to medications, if you're diabetic or you have other special problems, it's important to wear medical identification in the form of tags on a necklace or bracelet.

If you don't have a Medic-Alert bracelet, write out your own medical record, which is your own Vital Information Card. You could ask your nurse or pharmacist to help you prepare this card. It should contain the following information:

Your name, address, and phone number
Your doctor's name and phone number
Your illness or condition
Your medications, doses prescribed, and how often
   you take them
Your allergies or special medical problems
Whom to call in case of emergency

Carry this Vital Information Card with you at all times.

As we've said before, but will say again, if you pass out, you want the best and quickest help possible. If you're unable to speak, you want people to know if you're allergic to penicillin. If you have a seizure disorder, it should say so on the card. If you carry medication that will correct a reaction you may be having, put that on the card as well. If you wear contact lenses, write that on your card.

If you're a regular member of a senior center or an organization that meets regularly, talk to the social worker and put your health information and problems on the record so that they'll have necessary information at their fingertips if needed.

If your parent is in a senior citizens' center and can't speak on her own behalf for some reason, let the center know if your parent has a heart condition or some other serious medical problem. Provide them with the name of the doctor, and tell them what medication she is on. Tell your parent that you're giving the center this information so that they can help her if she needs it. Be careful not to embarrass your parent by giving out private information that the center does not need.

Long-term Precautions

On a long-term basis, it's also a good idea—no matter your age—to start keeping a medication diary. Buy a good, sturdy notebook or hardcover book that will last.

Keep a permanent record that starts with the date, names your condition, and lists the medications you're using. Make sure to write down the amount, how often, and how long you take each medication. If you have any side effects or allergic reactions, write them into the diary. If your doctor changes the dosage, write the change into your diary. Write down your response or reactions to the drugs. Each time you visit any doctor or health maintenance organization, take along your medication diary.

Jot down your over-the-counter drugs in this diary as well. Note how often you use the drug and what the effect is. Here's an example of how you could set up your medication diary:

DATE	CONDITION	PRESCRIPTION	AMOUNT	DIRECTIONS	REACTIONS
10/1/86	Bronchitis	Tetracycline	250 mg	PO QID FOR 7 DAYS/Do Not Take With Dairy Products	Cramps

Make sure to leave space to write comments. Under this entry, for instance, you want to have room to write down all your reactions to the medicine, whether the doctor changed the dose or the medication, and how you responded to the new prescription.

Looking at the medication diary, you should be able to see the date and year of each prescription, how long you took it, and how you reacted to it. Who can remember, after all, what antibiotic you were given in 1978 and how you reacted to it then? If you have it written down in your medication diary, you'll be able to tell a new physician whether you've been on a particular medication before and how you responded to it. If you don't have it written down, you won't be able to tell him that you did have it and it made you feel dizzy and sick. (Was it *that* medication or another one?)

When a doctor asks you if you ever had sulfacytine before, for instance, and you know that you had it two years ago and it made your muscles ache and gave you a skin rash, he has something to go on. If you don't know, it's like starting all over again. A doctor is taking the risk of exposing you to something you had an intolerance to before, but you may react even more seriously to it this time. Keeping records makes you a better patient and an informed and intelligent ally in your own health care.

WHEN YOU'RE TRAVELING

Make sure to tell your doctor and your pharmacist before you leave on a trip and ask them to tell you, based on the details of your specific health history, what you should take along in case of emergency.

Along with the additional medications they suggest, take along your Vital Information Card and the day-to-day medications you'll need for the duration of your travels. Take an extra week's supply in case you're delayed for some reason.

If you must take a certain medication on a daily basis, carry it with you—in your purse or briefcase—when you travel by airplane. Don't take the chance of leaving it in a suitcase that gets sent to Toronto instead of Buffalo.

If you're planning to travel to Europe, the Middle East, Asia, South America, or anywhere else overseas, ask your doctor to help you make plans as far ahead of time as possible.

What extra medications should you take along for possible problems of constipation?

What about diarrhea? Sometimes with a change of diet, you will get a slight case of diarrhea from normal (and harmless) bacterial changes in the food you're eating. If this happens to you, Pepto-Bismol should take care of it. If the diarrhea persists, however, or if it is accompanied by chills, fever, or abdominal cramps, then you should see a doctor rather than trying to medicate it yourself.

What do you need to know about the interactive effects of the medicines you're taking along?

What sort of health record should you bring along just in case you need to be treated overseas? What does your doctor recommend?

What should you do if you lose or run out of your medication for any reason on the trip?

Remember that if you're in a foreign country, you have no Medicare coverage. Also, if you're traveling with someone else, remember to tell your traveling companion(s) where you carry your list of vital information. Tell him where you keep your heart pills and any other critical medication he might need in case of an emergency. Tell him if you have any special condition or allergies.

Eventually, probably the only medical record you'll need to carry along with you when traveling or even going to the grocery store is something the size of a credit card that has all vital medical information about you written on it. Recently, Blue Cross/Blue Shield of Maryland announced plans to introduce just such a laser-encoded card to its subscribers in Columbia, Maryland. The card can carry a person's entire medical history on its surface, including X rays, vaccination records, and EKGs. The card, which depends on laser optic technology, can hold up to eight hundred pages of medical information, including a digitized personal photograph and an explanation of insurance coverage. It also contains all information on allergies, medications, dosages, and special problems.

These cards, or something like them, will probably be used widely by doctors, dentists, health-main-

tenance organizations, and hospitals. You'll have a
Vital Information Card that will have more vital statistics on it than you'd ever care to remember, and all
you will have to do when you see a new doctor is
hand over your ''credit card'' (having checked first
to make sure that all the information is correct!).

In the meantime, however, for the next ten or fifteen
years at least, the job will still depend on your own
record-keeping skills and your attention to the details
at hand.

WHEN YOU'RE ENTERING THE HOSPITAL

If you are going into the hospital for surgery or
for a period of observation, take along all the prescriptions and nonprescription medicines you've been
taking. Show them to your doctor or nurse and ask
them to review them with you. If you haven't
had time to collect them at home, ask a friend
to bring them in, or make a list of them for review.

Let your doctor and nurses know your allergies. Make
sure that they're written on your chart.

While you're in the hospital, find out what medications you're being given. Write down the names of
the drugs and ask what they're for. If a nurse wakes
you up to give you medication, ask her what the pill
is and what you're taking it for before you swallow
it. Most likely the medication has been ordered for
you, and it is your medicine, but find out anyway. If
you don't recognize the medication and its purpose,
refuse to take it until you are satisfied with answers
as to why it will benefit you. If you don't want to
take the medication in question, you don't have to.
It's your body, your life, and your health. Don't
be bullied or intimidated. You have every right to

make choices about what to do in your own best
interest.

WHEN YOU'RE LEAVING THE HOSPITAL

When you're leaving the hospital, you'll probably be
given one or more prescriptions to have filled. Make
sure you have whatever prescription orders you need to
take along.

Usually a nurse will sit down with you and go over
all the medications with you as part of your discharge.
Ask the nurse for the generic name and the brand name
of each medication. Make sure you know the purpose
of the drug, the dosage, how often you're supposed to
take it, and the manner in which you're supposed to
take it. Ask about side effects to expect and side effects
to report. Ask about which foods and beverages you
should avoid.

Check with the doctor or nurse about what to do about
medications you were taking at home before you came
into the hospital. It may be that you're not supposed to
take what you were taking before, but that should be
clarified.

When you get home, have someone go over all your
medicines with you. Clean out your medicine cabinet
and throw away medications that you're not supposed
to be taking anymore. You won't take the wrong medicine if it's not in your cabinet.

TIPS FOR CARE-GIVERS

Ask your spouse, parent, friend, or relative if they understand what medicines they're taking and why.

If they're confused or unable to comprehend their
treatment for any reason, find out yourself. Get a list
of their medicines and find out how much and how

often they're supposed to take them. Watch for changes or any worsening of their condition. Ask who is coordinating the medicines and make sure that person knows everything she needs to know about the patient's medical history, allergies, and drug history. Make sure that no one adds medicines without a consultation. Find out if there is cooperation (at the health-maintenance organization, hospital, or institution) among the nurses, doctors, pharmacists, and nutritionists. Are they working as an interdisciplinary team?

If you can, write up a drug history on your family member or friend. Get help in developing medication schedules and systems for medication taking to aid the person with a memory loss or physical disability.

If They're Moving into a Nursing Home

If you have a friend or relative moving into a nursing home, act as an advocate. Remember to be aware at all times of what medications that person is receiving—how much and how often. Ask questions and pay attention to what is being done so that the staff of the nursing home will be fully aware that someone is observing the treatment of that person. There are some excellent nursing homes, but even at excellent homes there may be a tendency to overmedicate patients.

If you have a friend or loved one in a nursing home who suddenly seems groggy, confused, or sedated, find out if they've been given a new medication. Are they being drugged to keep them quiet? You have the right, if not the duty, to intervene on behalf of the person who is sick.

Remember that if a person is groggy and can't walk, she won't be using her legs and arms or getting any good exercise. If patients don't use their muscles, those muscles may wither and they could end up confined in a wheelchair. If they try to walk when they're heavily sedated, they may end up breaking a leg or a hip.

Intervene on Their Behalf

If you are taking care of a friend or relative in a nursing home or in the hospital, feel free to talk to that person's physician about his treatment plan and about his medication. If you are the responsible relative, you usually have the right to request medication or to refuse medication on behalf of your impaired kin. If you think medication is making your loved one sick, make sure it's changed. Five percent of all older people are living in nursing homes at any one time—and for them, it's like entering a totally new world. As many reports have indicated, people in nursing homes lose their sense of entitlement and are often treated as if they have no rights—that is, no right to question their doctors, no right to refuse treatment, no right to their own opinions. In fact, they have all those rights. It's often critical for nursing-home patients to have you advocate on their behalf, to have you know all the prescription and nonprescription drugs they're taking, and to have you know the names and treatment plans of all the doctors involved. It's also important to know who is acting as pharmacist for the patient and who is in charge of coordinating the treatment plan. Get to know the caretakers and the professionals and keep the communication flowing.

A LOOK AT THE FUTURE

It seems clear by now that the vast majority of drug problems that older people face can, indeed, be remedied with good information and careful preventative action.

As our population ages, it's increasingly important

to solve the critical problems created for older people and the society by the medications that have been prescribed for them. The hundreds of thousands of illnesses, injuries, hospitalizations, and deaths that older people experience because of their medications make this a drug crisis of epidemic proportions. Certainly, in terms of health-care costs and life-and-death matters, this is as severe a drug crisis as this country has ever faced.

FDA Commissioner Frank E. Young, M.D., said at a news conference on drug misuse, "The toll in mental disorientation, in physical effects, and even in terms of life and death, may be just as great when a seventy-year-old woman takes her blood pressure medicine improperly as when her grandson smokes marijuana or takes a street drug."

By the year 2050, one out of every eight people will be seventy-five or older, and it is estimated that by then, older people will be purchasing 50 percent of all medications. Dr. Young points out that in many cases, men and women who have spent most of their lifetimes not taking even an aspirin will become the men and women who require several drugs for blood pressure and/or glaucoma and/or arthritis and/or diabetes. These people need to be educated about drug use. They need information on medicines, and they need to understand the importance of that information. Additionally, doctors, nurses, pharmacists, and other health-care professionals must become more aware of the effects of medications on older people. Without this vital awareness and a campaign for the prevention of adverse reactions to drugs, this country will see a crisis in health care that reaches unmanageable proportions.

Afterword

In many ways, medicine is an everyday story, and it's one that affects all of us directly or indirectly at some time or other. Usually, it's a story without real drama. But what's surprising is how, when mistakes are made, it almost instantly contains all the pathos and tragedy of high drama.

Medicines are still mysterious, still beyond our full understanding. They're not totally unlike the magic potions brewed by sorcerers of old. Poof! They make the sickness go away! Poof! They cast a spell that makes the sickness worse.

If not used properly, medicines have the power to make us lose our memory, make us stumble, or make us fall. They put us into a deep sleep, like Snow White's, or cause our faces and eyes to swell to the point where both Beauty and the Beast would cry for us. Sometimes a drug shakes us to our toes. Other times it clears the shakes away. A minute quantity modifies our system and corrects it. Trace elements that are missing are magically replaced, giving us a renewed peace and calm.

No matter how little we know, we can learn enough to make the medications we use work for us. What we have to remember is that, in fact, the use of drugs is not an abstraction. It's real and very concrete. It's not only the infirm, the crippled, the people in nursing homes or hospitals we're concerned about when we discuss the importance of knowing about and managing our medications. It's an issue of importance to all of us.

Life holds many options. The nature of experience can vary tremendously throughout one's life span. Old age should bring with it a continuation of the threads woven through our histories, along with the fun of the spontaneous or unexpected feeling, new insights and challenges. It should not bring with it an expectation of deficits, but rather an embracement of all that has been gained and can still be enjoyed.

Geriatrics has led medical professionals to look at the quality of life in old age as a critical component of any medical decision. It's a discipline that has led to seeing older patients as people with an interest in living well and living fully. It emphasizes doing what is possible to make each day more comfortable and complete without jeopardizing the pleasures of being alive. If an eighty-nine-year-old man wants to have a quadruple bypass so that he can live longer and better, then geriatricians support that decision, and well may have the pleasure of seeing that same patient get his gallbladder taken out at the age of ninety-seven, and continue to work every day at the age of ninety-nine.

If a ninety-two-year-old with cancer of the kidney wants to have her kidney removed because she can't bear the pain, then the geriatrician has been the one to insist on the operation when other doctors refused because the patient was "too old."

In the same way, geriatricians may be the only doctors who regularly refuse to give a medication when they believe it will interfere with the quality of their patients' existence. They know from experience that giving a medication to achieve some long-term physiological benefit is just not worth the sacrifice of making the older person impotent, confused, or miserable.

Every day, the clarity of our observations, explorations, and interactions are dramatically affected by the way we feel. Our intellectual quests, our spirit, humor, and sense of self are diminished when we have stomach cramps or feel irritable from the effects of medication. The small pleasures of being alive are modified as well. If I am dizzy and you are nauseated, we're not going to have much fun having lunch together. If my vision is blurred, if my skin is itching from a severe rash, or if I have a disturbing tremor in my arm, I'm not going to think about the nature of existence, let alone the magic of the world around me when I go on my morning walk.

The essence of who we are has to matter to us no matter how old we get. Everytime we take a medication, we have to ask why we need it and whether it will be a beneficial addition to our well-being. Our alertness and commitment to our own optimum health will invest in the future and help us live fully in the present.

APPENDIX

Patient Checklists and Records

ASK YOUR DOCTOR AND YOUR PHARMACIST*

☐ What is the name of this medication? (Ask for the brand name and the generic name.)

☐ What is it supposed to do for me? How does it work?

☐ Are there alternatives to this medication? For instance, could I change my diet or my life-style instead of taking this medication?

☐ How and when should I take it?

☐ Should I take this with food and liquids or on an empty stomach?

☐ Are there any foods or beverages I should avoid?

☐ Are there any foods or beverages I should add to my diet because of this medication?

☐ Are there any side effects I should expect?

☐ If I get any of these side effects, what should I do?

☐ Are there any adverse reactions I should watch out for?

☐ Will this medicine have any effect on my other medicines? Will they mix well?

*These instructions are reprinted with permission from Elder-Ed, the University of Maryland School of Pharmacy, 636 West Lombard Street, Baltimore, Maryland 21201.

- [ ] How would you suggest that I schedule taking my medicine?
- [ ] Is there anything I need to change in my life-style or be aware of when I take this drug?
- [ ] How long will I have to take this drug?
- [ ] Is there a good generic substitute for it at a lower cost?
- [ ] Do you have any written information on this drug that I could read?
- [ ] When should I contact you or see you again?

REMEMBER: If you don't understand what your doctor is saying, ask him to repeat it. If you can't hear him, say so. If you can't read the written instructions, tell him. If the type is too small for you to read on your prescription, ask your pharmacist to write it in *large* print.

If you start feeling sick, dizzy, confused, or crazy after you've started taking a medication, call your doctor immediately.

WHAT TO DO WITH YOUR MEDICINES*

- [ ] Always take medicine as directed.
- [ ] Make a schedule and mark when you take the medicine.
- [ ] Always check against directions.
- [ ] Do *not* hesitate to call your doctor if any of the following occurs:
    - nausea
    - stomach upset
    - light-headedness
    - any other unwanted effect from your medicine

*Reprinted with permission from The Parke-Davis Center for the Education of the Elderly, and Elder-Health Program, University of Maryland School of Pharmacy, 20 North Pine Street, Baltimore, Maryland 21201.

* the medicine does not do what you expected
☐ Store the medicine correctly. (Your pharmacist will suggest the right place.)
☐ Do *not* keep your medicines longer than is necessary.
☐ Do *not* "save" your medicine for use at some other time.
☐ Do *not* "share" your medicine with a friend or neighbor.
☐ *Do* refill your prescription as your doctor indicates.

COMBINATIONS TO AVOID!*

DON'T MIX THESE *Over-the-Counter Medications*	WITH THESE *Prescription Medications*
Aspirin or similar pain pills	Blood thinners
Antacids	Blood thinners Nerve pills Sleeping pills Heart pills Pills for parkinsonism Seizure pills
Certain laxatives, alcohol, vitamin C	Blood thinners
Low-sodium diet	Effervescent Antacids Laxatives Pain preparations

*This format was created by the Parke-Davis Center for the Education of the Elderly, and the Elder-Health Program at the University of Maryland School of Pharmacy, 20 North Pine Street, Baltimore, Maryland 21201.

PERSONAL MEDICATION RECORD*

NAME:_____

ADDRESS:_____

DOCTOR'S NAME:_____

DOCTOR'S TELEPHONE NUMBER:_____

PHARMACY NAME (AND PHARMACIST):_____

PHARMACIST'S TELEPHONE NUMBER:_____

IN CASE OF EMERGENCY, CALL (NAME):_____

AT (PHONE NUMBER):_____

Conditions I am being treated for:_____
_____
_____
_____

I have the following allergic reactions or drug sensitivities:

_____
_____
_____

*Reprinted with permission by The Parke-Davis Center for the Education of the Elderly, and the Elder-Health Program at the University of Maryland School of Pharmacy, 20 North Pine Street, Baltimore, Maryland 21201.

Prescription Medicines I Am Taking Regularly or as Needed:

NAME OF MEDICINE	DOSE	DIRECTIONS	REACTIONS

Nonprescription Medicines I Am Taking Regularly or as Needed:

NAME OF MEDICINE	DOSE	DIRECTIONS	REACTIONS

WEEKLY MEDICATION CALENDAR

DATES: From _____ to _____

At the beginning of the week, fill in the name of the medication and the times for you to take it. Each time you take a medication, put a check beside the time you took it.

	NAME OF MEDICINE	DOSE	TIME	TIME	TIME	TIME
SUNDAY						
MONDAY						
TUESDAY						
WEDNESDAY						
THURSDAY						
FRIDAY						
SATURDAY						

COMMONLY PRESCRIBED DRUGS THAT ARE AVAILABLE GENERICALLY

The following table, compiled by the FDA and published in the FDA *Consumer*, lists the fourteen most often prescribed drugs that are available generically. If you are taking one of these drugs under a brand name, it may save you money to buy its generic form instead. Ask your physician and pharmacist about it. If your doctor doesn't have a sound medical reason for preferring a brand name drug, he'll probably write a generic prescription for you. Many other drugs besides these have generic equivalents, so whenever you get a new prescription, remember to ask if it's available generically.

GENERIC NAME	COMMONLY PRESCRIBED BRAND NAMES	PURPOSE OF DRUG
Ampicillin	Amcill Omnipen Polycillin Principen	To fight infection (antibiotic)
Tetracycline	Achromycin V Panmycin Sumycin Tetracyn	To fight infection (antibiotic)
Acetaminophen/codeine	Tylenol with Codeine	To relieve pain, fever, and cough
Hydrochlorothiazide	Esidrix HydroDIURIL Oretic	For hypertension and swelling of the legs (diuretic)

GENERIC NAME	COMMONLY PRESCRIBED BRAND NAMES	PURPOSE OF DRUG
Penicillin V-K	Pen. Vee K V-Cillin K Veetids	To fight infection (antibiotic)
Chlordiaze-poxide hydrochloride	Librium	To relieve anxiety and tension
Propoxyphene hydrochloride, aspirin, phenacetin, and caffeine	Darvon Compound-65	To relieve pain (analgesic)
Erythromycin stearate	Erythrocin Stearate	To fight infection (antibiotic)
Amitriptyline hydrochloride	Elavil Endep	To relieve symptoms of depression
Diphen-hydramine hydrochloride	Benadryl	Antihistamine (also for motion sickness and parkinsonism)
Meclizine hydrochloride	Antivert	To control nausea and vomiting, dizziness, and motion sickness
Chlorothiazide	Diuril	For hypertension

GENERIC NAME	COMMONLY PRESCRIBED BRAND NAMES	PURPOSE OF DRUG
		and edema (diuretic)
Erythromycin ethyl succinate	E.E.S.	To fight infection (antibiotic)
Digoxin	Lanoxin	To treat heart failure and atrial fibrillation

Because older age brings changes in the functioning and structure of the body that may alter drug action, drug treatment must be accompanied by very careful consideration of drugs and dosage, schedules along with the individual's health and tolerances. According to James Long's *The Essential Guide to Prescription Drugs*, the following drugs should be carefully considered in light of their potential adverse reactions for people sixty-five and older.*

Drugs best avoided by the elderly because of increased possibility of adverse reactions:

antacids (high sodium)   indomethacin (Indocin)
barbiturates   phenacetin
cycloposphamide   phenylbutazone
  (Cytosian)   (Butazolidin)

---

*This list has been reprinted with permission from *The Essential Guide to Prescription Drugs: What You Need to Know for Safe Drug Use* by James W. Long, M.D. (New York: Harper and Row, 1985). Please note that while this is a verbatim reprint, many doctors might disagree with the complete list of drugs to be avoided. Estrogen, for instance, is recommended by many doctors, as is Parnate. Conversely, some drugs may have been omitted that some doctors might consider problematic.

diethylstibestrol
estrogens

tetracyclines
tranylcypromine (Parnate)

Drugs that should be used by the elderly in reduced dosages until full effect has been determined:

anticoagulants (oral)
antidepressants
antidiabetic drugs
antihistamines
antihypertensives
barbiturates
beta-blockers
colchicine (Colbenemid)
cortisonelike drugs
digitalis preparations
diuretics (all types)
ephedrine
epinephrine
fenoprofen
haloperidol (Haldol)
ibuprofen (Motrin)

isoetharine (Brethine)
metoprolol (Lopressor)
nalidixic acid
naproxen (Naprosyn, Anaprox)
narcotic drugs
prazosin (Minipress)
propranolol (Inderal)
pseudoephedrine (Sudafed)
quinidine
sleep inducers (hypnotics)
sulindac (Clinoril)
terbutaline
thyroid preparations
tolmetin (Tolectin)

Drugs that may cause confusion and behavioral disturbances in the elderly:

amantadine
antidepressants
antidiabetic drugs
antihistamines
atropine and drugs containing belladonna
barbiturates
benzodiazepines
carbamazepine
cimetidine
digitalis preparations
dihydroergotoxine

L-dopa
meprobamate
methocarbamol
methyldopa (Aldomet)
narcotic drugs
pentazocine (Talwin)
phenytoin (Dilantin)
primidone
reserpine
sedatives
sleep inducers (hypnotics)
sulindac (Clinocil)

diuretics   thiothixene
fenoprofen   tranquilizers (mild)
ibuprofen (Motrin, Advil)   trihexyphenidyl

Drugs that may cause orthostatic hypotension in the elderly:
antidepressants   sedatives
antihypertensives   tranquilizers
diuretics (all types)   vasodilators
phenothiazines

Drugs that may cause constipation and/or retention of urine in the elderly:
amantadine   epinephrine
androgens   isoetharine
antidepressants   narcotic drugs
anti-parkinsonism drugs   phenothiazines
atropinelike drugs   terbutaline
dihydroergotoxine

Drugs that may cause loss of bladder control (urinary incontinence) in the elderly:
diuretics (all types)   sleep inducers (hypnotics)
sedatives   tranquilizers (mild)

Checklist:

FOR THE CARETAKERS OF AN ELDERLY FAMILY MEMBER OR FRIEND*

☐ Name of the patient's main doctor:_____
☐ Name of the patient's other doctors, including dentists, gynecologists, ophthalmologists, podiatrists, psychiatrists, or psychologists:

_____

☐ Name of the doctor who has agreed to coordinate the medicine plan of the patient. This doctor should be aware of *every* medication the patient is taking. (Is he?)_____

☐ Name of the pharmacy the patient uses:_____
☐ Name of the pharmacist in charge of the patient's records:

_____

☐ *All* the prescription drugs the patient is taking, the purpose of those drugs, how often or when the medication is supposed to be taken, and how much of it is supposed to be taken each time (e.g., one teaspoon, one pill):

NAME OF THE DRUG:	ITS PURPOSE:	HOW OFTEN:	HOW MUCH:
_____	_____	_____	_____
_____	_____	_____	_____
_____	_____	_____	_____
_____	_____	_____	_____

*This list was compiled chiefly from materials prepared by the Parke-Davis Center for the Education of the Elderly, and the Elder-Health Program at the University of Maryland School of Pharmacy.

☐ *All* the nonprescription (over-the-counter) drugs the patient is taking, including antacid tablets, cold medications, aspirin, laxatives, vitamins, and cough syrups—and how often they're taken:

_____
_____
_____

☐ Go over this list with the coordinating doctor. Is there anything on this list that should come off it? Are any of these medications contra-indicated? Could they be a bad mix for the patient?

☐ When the patient receives a new drug, ask the physician or the pharmacist what the medication should do for the patient. Is it supposed to stop diarrhea, for instance? Is it going to ease the pain but make the patient sleepy or groggy? What side effects should you expect from the medication? What is a normal range of reactions?

☐ Go over the name of the medication with the physician and the pharmacist. Confirm how to administer the medication, how often it should be taken, whether it should be taken with or without food. Ask how long this medication will be necessary.

☐ Can you read the label? Are the instructions clear? If the label says "before meals," does this mean immediately before meals, one hour or two hours before meals? If the doctor writes down "as needed" on the prescription, find out what he means by that. What are the symptoms that indicate the medication is needed. Don't assume you know. Ask.

☐ If the patient's physical or mental condition changes after he begins a new medication, call the doctor or pharmacist immediately and find out what to do. Most likely, the medication will be the source of this change.

☐ Although the patient may be bedridden, do *not* keep the medications by the bed if any children or grand-children come into the room. Don't keep sedatives or tranquilizers near the bed, either. The patient may be sleepy or confused and duplicate a pill he's al-ready taken. (The best place to keep medications is in a cool, dry place. Don't keep them near a radiator or in the bathroom.)

☐ Avoid giving tablets or capsules while the patient is lying down. Always give medicines with plenty of water. It helps them dissolve quickly.

☐ Avoid chewable tablets. They can interfere with dentures or be difficult to chew. Chewable tablets should *not* be swallowed whole.

☐ If necessary, tablets and capsules may be crushed or mixed into a spoonful of applesauce to make them easier to swallow. If you want to do this, check with the pharmacist first. Mix the medicine immediately before you are ready to give it to the patient. (Don't prepare this ahead of time.) Long-acting tablets should not be crushed.

☐ Talk to the patient's pharmacist or physician before selecting any over-the-counter medicine or ointment for the patient.

☐ Wash your hands after you've applied any medicinal ointments. Remember that these ointments work by

soaking through the skin. Wear gloves or use gauze
to apply ointment to any infected area of the skin.

☐ Don't switch from a liquid medication to a tablet
without discussing it first with the pharmacist or
doctor. The dosage may be different and may have
a different effect on the patient.

☐ If your family member or friend is going home from
the hospital or the nursing home, review medications
with the physician. The patient may have left home
with several drugs and be coming back with several
new ones. Which ones should the patient take? Which
ones should he or she disregard? What medication
plan will work best for what the patient is receiving?

☐ Don't assume that you know *why* the patient is feeling bad. Just because you feel a certain way when
you have a headache, that doesn't mean your friend
or relative is experiencing the same thing. He or she
may be having an appendicitis attack, for all you
know. Call the doctor.

☐ If your relative or friend tells you that he is tired,
aching, hurting, confused, dizzy—or that his stomach hurts, *listen carefully to the complaint*. Don't
assume that this person is just getting a little fuzzy
or hypochondriacal because of old age. It very well
may be that he's having a bad reaction to medication
or is seriously ill. Ask questions, and if there's any
doubt in your mind that this symptom could involve
illness or medication, call the doctor.

For Further Reference

About Your Medicines. The United States Pharmacopeial Convention, Inc., 12601 Twin Brook Parkway, Rockville, Maryland 20862.

This consumer's drug reference book provides information on over two thousand of the most commonly used prescription and over-the-counter medications. It is very clearly organized and advises you as to what to tell your doctor *before* using each medicine, how to use the medicine properly, what special medical precautions to take, what side effects are common and rare, what interactions with other drugs should be avoided, as well as what side effects may occur if you take a particular medicine for a long period of time. It also tells you how to store the drugs and informs you about what may happen to your body after you stop using a particular medicine for a long period of time. Published by the nonprofit organization that sets the official standards of strength, quality, and purity for drugs sold in the United States, this book provides an excellent reference for people interested in effectively managing their own medications.

Drug Evaluations, *Sixth Edition* American Medical Assn., 535 North Dearborn Street, Chicago, Illinois.

This reference provides complete and reliable information on more than 1,900 prescription and nonprescription drugs. Designed as an aid for physicians, it is also helpful for patients. It's very clearly organized and written, with tables for reference. Unlike the PDR, this book evaluates and compares drugs within classes and recommends certain drugs and regimes over others. If you want to be thoroughly informed, this book would be a valuable part of your drug reference library. It might turn out to be the mainstay.

Joe Graedon's The New People's Pharmacy #3; Drug Breakthroughs of the 80's, Joe Graedon and Theresa Graedon, New York: Bantam Books.

The People's Pharmacy, New York: St. Martin's Press,

The People's Pharmacy #2, Graedon Enterprises, Inc., PO Box 31788, Raleigh, North Carolina 27622.

Joe and Theresa Graedon's practical, down-to-earth discussions about medicines are fun and informative. These books are not thorough drug dictionaries, but they're packed with useful information on many commonly used drugs, side effects and dangerous drug interactions. They are also organized according to subject matter and provide a context and approach to particular conditions. *The People's Pharmacy* contains information on allergies, asthma, contraception, and drug interactions. *The People's Pharmacy-2* discusses arthritis therapies, vitamins, special problems with drugs used by older people, booby traps in over-the-counter medicines, and drugs used most effectively to treat insomnia. *Joe Graedon's The New People's Pharmacy* includes a look at the miracles of all the new medications on the market today, their dangers and alternatives; medicines for your heart and hypertension; recent information about ulcer medications; and some behind-the-scenes ''shop'' talk about scandals in the drug industry and the FDA.

* * *

Long, James W. *The Essential Guide to Prescription Drugs*. New York, Harper and Row, 1977.
This book by Dr. James Long provides a comprehensive, well-organized, and thoughtful analysis of brand name and generic drugs. It tells available dosage forms and strengths, the availability of the drug by generic name, how the drug works, and what it should do. It lets you know what side effects are common and should be expected and what side effects are rare and unexpected. It tells you when *not* to take a drug and when to inform your doctor before taking it. It also lists precautions to observe while taking the drug and itemizes each product's interactions with other drugs. The back of the book contains tables of drug information that are excellent references.

The Medical Letter on Drugs and Therapeutics. The Medical Letter, Inc., 56 Harrison Street, New Rochelle, New York 10801.

The Medical Letter gives short but succinct reviews of new drugs and updates on old drugs. It tells you how a drug works, what indications are needed for its use, and the expected results of its usage. It tells you the pharmacokinetics of a drug, its clinical trials and adverse reactions. It compares each drug to other drugs, discusses it, and gives you the cost. This letter is one of the best sources of information based on clinical practice and is a great educational reference. It's no harder to read than the *Physicians' Desk Reference* and has the added benefit of putting information on each drug into perspective as well as coming to conclusions on its usage. One doctor, who said she depends on *The Medical Letter*, called it "the Ralph Nader of medications."

Physicians' Desk Reference (PDR), Oradell, N.J.: Medical Economics Company, Inc.

The *PDR* is a complete standard reference for physicians. The book is quite thorough in relating side effects and information on dosage, but it presents information provided by drug companies without giving the consumer an analysis or a broader perspective on each drug. Often it's hard to find what you're looking for, since the bulk of information is arranged by pharmaceutical manufacturer, not by the drug. However, one advantage, if you want to go through the effort, is that you can identify your pills by looking at color photographs of capsules and tablets. While the PDR can sometimes be a valuable reference, it is dense in medical terminology. If you have a medical background or a great deal of persistence when it comes to researching information, you will find it helpful.

The Pill Book, by Silverman, Dr. Harold, New York: Bantam Books, Inc.

This small and compact book is well organized, clear, and easy to read. The information is brief but lists each drug by both its generic and its brand name, tells what it's prescribed for, and gives possible side effects, cautions, and warnings, along with helpful general and special information. A section with color photographs of pills will help you identify your particular drug. This book would be good to take with you if you're traveling; since it's small and reliable, it's an excellent reference to have on the road.

Worst Pills Best Pills: The Older Adult's Guide to Avoiding Drug-Induced Death or Illness, by Sidney M. Wolfe, M.D., Lisa Fugate, Elizabeth P. Hulstrand, Laurie E. Kamimoto, Public Citizen Health Research Group. Washington, D.C. Public Citizen Health Research Group, 1988.

* * *

This large and important book spells out the risks and benefits of the 287 most commonly used drugs for older people. It names 104 drugs commonly prescribed for older adults that should *not* be used by older adults because safer alternative drugs are available. They list these drugs under a DO NOT USE heading and name their safer alternatives. Printed in large type, this book is well organized and easy to understand.

References

Although this book is based primarily on personal interviews with physicians, pharmacists, nurses, patients, scientists, and gerontologists, I've also used the journal articles and books listed here to supplement that information, to add and confirm facts and technical details, and to provide a broader framework for my understanding. If you want to follow up on a particular subject or reference in greater depth, the following can serve as useful guides.

1. AN OVERVIEW—AGING AND THE USE OF MEDICINE

The British Medical Journal. Volume 290, 22 June 1985.

Butler, Robert N., M.D. *The Geriatric Patient.* Edited by William Reichel. New York: HP Publishing Co., 1978.

Butler, Robert N., M.D. *Why Survive? Being Old in America.* New York: Harper Colophon Books, 1975.

Butler, Robert N., M.D., and Alexander G. Bearn, M.D. *The Aging Process: Therapeutic Implications.* New York: Raven Press, 1985.

Calkins, Evan, M.D. "Residency Training in Geriatric Medicine—1984." Presented at the Eleventh Symposium on Medical Education, Committee on Medical Education, New York Academy of Medicine, 11 October 1984.

Cassells, Judith M., D.N.Sc., R.N., et al. "Student Choice of Baccalaureate Nursing Programs, Their Perceived Level of Growth and Development, Career Plans, and Transition into Practice: A Replication." *Journal of Professional Nursing,* May–June 1986.

Graedon, Joe, and Theresa Graedon. *Joe Graedon's The New People's Pharmacy*. New York: Bantam Books, 1985.

Gress, Lucille D., and Sister Rose Theres Bahr. *The Aging Person: A Holistic Perspective*. St. Louis: C. V. Mosby, 1983.

Kahn, Carol. *Beyond the Helix: DNA and the Quest for Longevity*. New York: Times Books, 1985.

Koch, Hugo. "Drug Utilization in Office Practice by Age and Sex of the Patient: National Ambulatory Medical Care Survey, 1980." U.S. Dept. of Health and Human Services, *Vital and Health Statistics of the National Center for Health Statistics*, no. 81 (July 26, 1982).

Krupat, Edward. "Physicians and Patients, A Delicate Balance." *Psychology Today*, November 1986.

Schneider, Edward L., M.D., and T. Franklin Williams, M.D. "Geriatrics and Gerontology: Imperatives in Education and Training." *Annals of Internal Medicine* 4, no. 3 (March 1986).

Sherman, Frederick T., and Leslie S. Libow. "Pharmacology and Medication." In *The Core of Geriatric Medicine*, edited by Leslie S. Libon and Frederick T. Sherman. St. Louis: C. V. Mosley, 1981.

Skinner, B. F., and M. E. Vaughan. *Enjoy Old Age*. New York: W. W. Norton, 1983.

Starr, Paul. *The Social Transformation of American Medicine*. New York: Basic Books, 1982.

Svarstadt, Bonnie. "Physician Patient Communication, and Patient Conformity and Medical Advice." In *The Growth of Bureaucratic Medicine*, edited by David Mechanic. New York: John Wiley & Sons, 1976.

Wolfe, Sidney M., Lisa Fugate, Elizabeth P. Hulstrand, Laurie E. Kamimoto, Public Citizen Health Research Group. *Worst Pills Best Pills: The Older Adult's Guide to Avoiding Drug-Induced Death or Illness*. Washington, D.C.: Public Citizen Health Research Group, 1988.

2. AM I SICK OR AM I JUST GETTING OLD?

Anderson, B., and E. Palmore. "Longitudinal Evaluation of Ocular Function." In *Normal Aging II*, edited by E. Palmore. Durham, N.C.: Duke University Press, 1974.

Bronson, Gail. "Aging Americans: Diversity of Older Set Underscored in Studies of Health and Welfare." *Wall Street Journal*, 29 October 1979.

Butler, Robert N., and Myrna L. Lewis. *Aging and Mental Health*. St. Louis: C. V. Mosby, 1977.

Freese, Arthur S. *The Brain and Aging: The Myths, the Facts*. Public Affairs Pamphlet, no. 591. New York: Public Affairs Committee, October 1985.

Frisch, Max. *Man in the Holocene*. Translated by G. Skelton. New York: Harcourt Brace Jovanovich, 1979.

Henig, Robin Marantz. *The Myth of Senility*. New York: Anchor Press/Doubleday, 1981.

Inoue, Yasushi. *Chronicle of My Mother*. Translated by Jean Oda Moy. Tokyo: Kodansha International, 1982.

Jarvik, L. F. "Diagnosis of Dementia in the Elderly: A 1980 Perspective." *Annual Review of Gerontology and Geriatrics*, 1980.

Kalish, Richard A. *Late Adulthood: Perspectives on Human Development*. Belmont, Calif.: Wadsworth, 1982.

Malcolm, M.T. "Alcohol and Drug Use in the Elderly Visited at Home." *The International Journal of the Addictions* 19 (4) (1984): 411–418.

Rowe, John W. M.D., and Richard Besdine, M.D., eds. *Health and Disease in Old Age*. Boston, Little, Brown, 1982.

Ruskin, Paul E. "A Piece of My Mind: Aging and Caring." *Journal of the American Medical Association* 250, no. 18 (November 11, 1983).

Sacks, Oliver. *Awakenings*. New York: E. P. Dutton, 1983.

——. *The Man Who Mistook His Wife for a Hat and Other Clinical Tales*. New York: Summit Books, 1986.

Thompson, Larry W., Ph.D., and Dolores Gallagher, Ph.D. "Depression and Its Treatment." *Aging*, no. 348 (1985).

U.S. Pharmacopeia. *Pharmacopeia of the United States of America*, 21st ed. (Rockland Maryland: U.S. Pharmacopeial Convention, Inc., 1985).

Verderber, Dolores. "Developmental Factors Affecting Health

of Adults." In *Essentials of Medical-Surgical Nursing; A Nursing Process Approach*, edited by Barbara C. Long, R.N., M.S.N., and Wilma J. Phipps, R.N., Pd.D., F.A.A.N. St. Louis: C. V. Mosby Co., 1985.

3. Rx: PRESCRIPTIONS FOR YOUR HEALTH

Allen, Marcia D. "Drug Therapy in the Elderly." *American Journal of Nursing*, August 1980.

American Association of Retired Persons. *Prescription Drugs: A Survey of Consumer Use, Attitudes and Behavior*. Washington, D.C., 1984.

Boykin, Stephen P., and Vincent de Paul Burkhart and Peter P. Lamy. "Drug Use in a Day Treatment Center." *The American Journal of Hospital Pharmacology* 35 (February 1978).

Butler and Bearne. *The Aging Process*.

Editors of *Consumer Guide*. with Nicola Giacona, Pharm. D. *People's Drug Guide*. New York: Beekman House, 1982.

Gordon, Alex, and Jules Saltman. *Know Your Medication: How to Use Over-the-Counter and Prescription Drugs*. Public Affairs Pamphlet no. 570. New York: Public Affairs Committee, February 1986.

Koch, Hugo. "Drugs Most Frequently Used in Office Practice: National Ambulatory Medical Care Survey, 1981." U.S. Dept. of Health and Human Services, *Vital and Health Statistics of the National Center for Health Statistics*, no. 89 (April 15, 1983).

Lamy, Peter, M.D. *Prescribing for the Elderly*. Littleton, MA.: PSG Publishing Co., 1980.

Libow, Leslie S. "General Concepts of Geriatric Medicine," in *The Core of Geriatric Medicine*.

——, and Frederick T. Sherman, "Pharmacology and Medication." *The Core of Geriatric Medicine*.

Long, James, M.D. *The Essential Guide to Prescription Drugs*. New York: Harper & Row, 1977.

Mintz, Morton. *The Therapeutic Nightmare*. Boston: By Prescription Only, 1967.

Silverman, Harold M., and Gilbert I. Simon. *The Pill Book*. 2d ed. New York: Bantam Books, 1979.

Wolfe, Sidney M., Lisa Fugate, Elizabeth P. Hulstrand, Laurie

E. Kamimoto, Public Citizen Health Research Group. *Worst Pills Best Pills: The Older Adult's Guide to Avoiding Drug-Induced Death or Illness*. Washington, D.C.: Public Citizen Health Research Group, 1988.

4. TAKING COMMAND OF YOUR PRESCRIPTIONS

Editors of Consumer Guide with Nicola Giacona, Pharm., D. *People's Drug Guide*. Beekman House, New York, 1982.

Gordon and Saltman. *Know Your Medication*.

Kepler, Ann and James, with William Swisher, M.D. *The After-50 Pharmacy*. Chicago: Contemporary Books, 1986.

Long. *The Essential Guide to Prescription Drugs*.

Physicians' Desk Reference. Edward R. Barnhart, Publisher. 40th edition. Oradell, N.J.: Medical Economics Company 1986.

Plant, Janet. "Educating the Elderly in Safe Medication Use." *Hospitals Journal of the American Hospital Association* 51 (April 16, 1977).

Robb, Caroline, with Janet Reynolds. *The Caregiver's Guide: Helping Older Relatives and Friends with Health and Safety*. Boston: Houghton Mifflin, 1991.

Siegelman, Stanley. "Scribbled Rx's by MD's Result in RPh Errors; Many Patients End Up with Wrong Medication." *American Druggist* 187(5)(1983):3.

U.S. Department of Health, Education and Welfare, National Institute on Drug Abuse. *Using Your Medicines Wisely: A Guide for the Elderly*. Chevy Chase, Md. 1977.

Weiman, Henry, M.D. "Avoid Common Pitfalls of Geriatric Prescribing." *Geriatrics* 41, no. 6 (June 1981).

5. CAUSES AND EFFECTS OF AGING—A PATH INTO THE FUTURE

Allen, Marcia D. "Drug Therapy in the Elderly." *American Journal of Nursing*, August 1980.

American Association of Colleges of Pharmacy, Geriatric Curriculum Project, Health Sciences Consortium. *Pharmacy Practice for the Geriatric Patient*. Carrboro, N.C., 1985.

Butler and Bearn. *The Aging Process.*

Finch, Caleb E. "New Questions About Steroids." *Journal of the American Geriatric Society* 34 (1986): 393–94.

Funcillo, Richard J. "Drug Therapy in the Elderly." *Clinical Pharmacology,* February 1987.

Gilchrest, Barbara A., and John W. Rowe. "The Biology of Aging." In *Health and Disease in Old Age*, edited by John W. Rowe, M.D., and Richard W. Besdine, M.D. Boston: Little, Brown, 1982.

Gioiella, Evelynn Clark, R.N., Ph.D. "The Aging Process—Physical Adaptations." *Nursing Care of the Aging Client.* Norwalk, Conn.: Appleton-Century-Crofts, 1985.

Hayflick, Leonard. "The Cellular Basis for Biological Aging." In *Handbook of the Biology of Aging*, edited by Caleb E. Finch and Leonard Hayflick. New York: Van Nostrand Reinhold, 1977.

Picozzi, A., and E. A. Neidle. "Geriatric Pharmacology for the Dentist, An Overview." *Dental Clinics of North America.* July 28, 1984.

Rowe and Besdine, *Health and Disease in Old Age.*

Schneider and Williams. "Geriatrics and Gerontology."

Wolford, Roy L. *Maximum Life Span.* New York: Avon Books, 1984.

6. HOW YOUR BODY RESPONDS TO DRUGS—SIDE EFFECTS, ALLERGIC REACTIONS, AND TOXIC REACTIONS

Avorn, Jerome, M.D. "Drug Use and Misuse: A Growing Concern for Older Americans." Statement to the Joint Hearing Before the Special Committee on Aging, U.S. House of Representatives, 28 June 1983.

Butler and Bearn. *The Aging Process.*

Graedon, Joe. *The People's Pharmacy.* New York: Avon Books, 1980.

Lamy, Peter P. "Patterns of Prescribing and Drug Use." In Butler and Bearn, *The Aging Process.*

Lamy, Peter P. "Appropriate and Inappropriate Drug Use in the Geriatrics Patient." *Pharmacy Practice for the Geriatric Pa-*

tient. The American Association of Colleges of Pharmacy, Health Sciences Consortium. Carrboro, N.C., 1985.

Pulliam, Charles C., and Ronald B. Stewart, "Adverse Drug Reactions in the Elderly," American Association of Colleges of Pharmacy, Health Sciences Consortium, *Pharmacy Practice for the Geriatric Patient.*

Rosenbaum, J., and M. Pollack. "Treatment-Emergent Incontinence with Lithium." *Journal of Clinical Psychiatry* 46 (October 1985):444–45.

Wade, Barbara and Amy Bowling. "Appropriate Use of Drugs by Elderly People." *Journal of Advanced Nursing* 11 (April 1986).

Williamson, J., and J. M. Chopin. "Adverse Reactions to Prescribed Drugs in the Elderly: A Multicenter Investigation." *Age and Aging*, September 1980.

7. POLYPHARMACY—YOUR BODY AS "DRUG CENTRAL"

Allen, Marcia D. "Drug Therapy in the Elderly."

American Association of Colleges of Pharmacy, Health Sciences Consortium. *Pharmacy Practice for the Geriatric Patient.*

Berkow, Robert, M.D., and John H. Talbot, M.D.D., eds. *The Merck Manual of Diagnosis and Therapy.* 13th ed. Rahway, N.J.: Merck, Sharp and Dohme, 1977.

Brenton, Myron. "Women and Abuse of Prescription Drugs." Public Affairs Pamphlet, no. 604. New York: Public Affairs Committee, July 1982.

Carruthers, George. "Clinical Pharmacology of Aging," *Fundamentals of Geriatric Medicine.* New York: Raven Press, 1983.

"Drug Use and Misuse: A Growing Concern for Older Americans." Statement to the Joint Hearing Before the Special Committee on Aging, U.S. House of Representatives, 28 June 1983.

Henning, Janet. "Drug Interactions: Two Are Not Always Better Than One. *Journal of Practical Nursing*, 1975.

Lieff, Dr. Jonathan D., M.D. Statement to the Joint Hearing before the Special Committee on Aging, U.S. House of Representatives, 28 June 1983.

Long. *The Essential Guide to Prescription Drugs.*

Zimney, Mrs. Rose. Statement to the Joint Hearing Before the Special Committee on Aging, U.S. House of Representatives, 28 June 1983.

8. DRUGS IN DISGUISE—FOOD, ALCOHOL, AND DRUG COMBINATIONS

Blakeslee, Sandra. "Nicotine: Harder to Kick Than Heroin." *The New York Times Magazine* Part 2, March 1987.

Brenton, Myron. "Women and Abuse of Prescription Drugs." Public Affairs Pamphlet, no. 604 New York: Public Affairs Committee, July 1982.

Butters, Nelson, and Jason Brandt. "The Continuity Hypothesis: The Relationship of Long-Term Alcoholism to the Wernicke-Korsakoff Syndrome." *Recent Advances in Alcoholism.* Vol. 2, New York: Plenum Press, 1985.

"Caution on Mushrooms." *Wellness Letter.* Newsletter of Nutrition, Fitness and Stress Management, University of California, Berkeley, pub. in association with the School of Public Health, July 1986.

DiCicco-Bloom, Barbara, et al. "The Homebound Alcoholic." *American Journal of Nursing*, February 1986.

Dobmeyer, David J., et al. "The Arrhythmogenic Effects of Caffeine in Human Beings." *New England Journal of Medicine* 308 (1983).

Goldstein, Richard. "Getting Real About Getting High: An Interview with Andrew Weil, M.D." *Village Voice*, 30 September 1986.

Graedon. *The New People's Pharmacy.*

Hartford, J. T., and T. Samaorajski. "Alcoholism in the Geriatric Population." *Journal of American Geriatric Society*, 30 January 1982.

Jacobson, Michael F. *The Complete Eater's Digest and Nutrition Scoreboard.* New York: Anchor Press/Doubleday, 1985.

Malcolm, M.T., M.D., M.R.C. Psych. "Alcohol and Drug Use in the Elderly Visited at Home." *The International Journal of the Addictions* 19, no. 4 (1984).

Pepper, Claude. Statement to the Subcommittee on Health and Long-Term Care, U.S. House of Representatives, 21 July 1983.

Scribner, Belding H. "Salt and Hypertension." *Journal of the American Medical Association* 250 (1983).

Space, Sharon. "The Elderly Alcoholic." *Passage* (Journal of Catholic Charities, Rockville Centre), January 1985.

"Substance Abuse in the Elderly." *Medical Aspects of Human Sexuality* 18, no. 8 (August 1984).

9. OVER-THE-COUNTER DRUGS—FADS AND FACTS

American Association of Retired Persons. *Prescription Drugs: A Survey of Consumer Use, Attitudes and Behavior.*

Brody, Jane. *Jane Brody's Nutrition Book.* New York: W. W. Norton, 1981.

Caroselli-Karinja, Marie, R.N., B.S.N. "Drug Abuse and the Elderly." *Journal of Psychosocial Nursing* 23, no. 6 (June 1985).

Editors of Consumer Guide. *The Vitamin Book.* New York: Simon & Schuster, 1979.

Graedon and Graedon. *The New People's Pharmacy.*

Harkness, Richard P., Ph.D. *OTC Handbook: What to Recommend and Why.* Oradell, N.J.: Medical Economics Books 1983.

Hecht, Annabel. "Medicine and the Elderly." *FDA Consumer*, HHHS Publication no. (FDA) 83-3138 (September 1983).

"Impaired Vision From Overuse of Nasal Spray." *Nurses' Drug Alert*, April 1986.

Inglefinger, Dr. Franz. *New England Journal of Medicine.*

Institute of Medicine, National Academy of Sciences. "Sleeping Pills, Insomnia and Medical Practice." Report of a Study. Washington, D.C., 1979.

Kaufman, Joel, et al. *Over-the-Counter Pills That Don't Work.* New York: Pantheon Books, 1983.

Kripke, Daniel F., M.D., et al. "Short and Long Sleep and Sleeping Pills: Is Increased Mortality Associated?" *Arch Gen Psychiatry* 36 (January 1979).

Mellinger, Glen D., Ph.D., et al. "Insomnia and Its Treatment." *Arch Gen. Psychiatry* 42 (March 1985).

Salzman, Carl. *Clinical Geriatric Psycho-Pharmacology.* New York: McGraw-Hill, 1984.

Sherman, Frederick T., and Leslie S. Libow. "Pharmacology and Medication."

Spencer, Roberta, and Doris Alexander. "Counseling Clients Regarding-Over-the-Counter Drug Use." *Journal of Community Health Nursing* 3, no. 1 (1986).

"The OTC/HBA Battleground," *Drug Topics*. April 1991.

10. YOUR SEXUALITY AND MEDICATION

Berger, Richard E., M.D., and Deborah Berger, M.S.W. "It May Not Be in Your Head—A Guide to Sexual Potency." Book proposal, 1986.

Brody, Jane E. "Personal Health: Whether to Replace Estrogen That's Lost During Menopause." *New York Times*, 17 April 1985.

——. "Prostate, Bane of Aging Men, Is Yielding to New Treatments." *New York Times*, 9 April 1985.

Butler, Robert N., M.D., and Myrna Lewis, A.C.S.W. *Love and Sex After Forty.* New York: Harper & Row, 1986.

——. *Love and Sex After Sixty: A Guide for Men and Women in Their Later Years.* New York: Harper & Row, 1976.

Coope, Jean M.D. *The Menopause.* New York: Arco, 1984.

Cutler, Winnifred Berg, Ph.D., et al. *Menopause.* New York: W. W. Norton, 1983.

Kinsey, Alfred, et al. *Sexual Behavior in the Human Male.* Philadelphia: W. B. Saunders, 1948.

——. *Sexual Behavior in the Human Female.* Philadelphia: W. B. Saunders, Co., 1953.

Leaf, Alexander, M.D. *Youth in Old Age.* New York: McGraw Hill, 1975.

Lobsenz, Norman M. "Sex After Sixty-five." Public Affairs Pamphlet no. 519, New York: Public Affairs Committee, May 1986.

Masters, William H., and Virginia E. Johnson. *Human Sexual Inadequacy.* Boston: Little, Brown & Company, 1970.

——. *Human Sexual Response.* Boston: Little, Brown & Company, 1966.

Long. *The Essential Guide to Prescription Drugs.*

Pesmen, Curtis, and the editors of *Esquire. How a Man Ages:*

Growing Older: What to Expect and What You Can Do About It. New York: Ballantine Books, 1984.

Pfeiffer, Eric, M.D. "Psychosomatic Aspects of Aging." *Aspects of Aging*. Philadelphia: Smith, Kline & French, 1985. Report no. 6, unit 1, 1985.

Stoppard, Dr. Miriam. *The Best Years of Your Life*. New York: Ballantine Books, 1987.

11. EXTENDING YOUR LIFE—FOLK REMEDIES, QUACK CURES, NUTRITION, AND EXERCISE

American Association of Retired Persons. *Pep Up Your Life: A Fitness Book for Seniors*, a pamphlet. Washington, D.C., 1985.

Blumberg, Jeffrey B. "Nutrient Requirements for the Healthy Elderly." *Contemporary Nutrition*. Vol. XI, No. 6 (1986).

Briley, Michael. "Staying Well: The $10 Billion Scandal." *Modern Maturity*, April–May 1985.

Butler, Robert N. *Why Survive?*

deVries, Herbert A., with Diane Hales. *Fitness After 50*. New York: Charles Scribner's Sons, 1974.

Fiatarone, Maria, M.D., et al. "Stimulation of Natural Killer Cell Activity by Beta-Endorphin and Interleukin-2 in Elderly Subjects." *Clinical Research* 35 (1987): 455A.

Frankel, Laurence J., and Betty Byrd Richard. *Be Alive as Long as You Live*. New York: Lippincott and Crowell, 1980.

Goleman, Daniel. "Relaxation: Surprising Benefits Detected." *The New York Times*, 13 May 1986.

Kart, Cary S., and Seamus P. Metress. *Nutrition, The Aged and Society*. Englewood Cliffs, N.J.: Prentice-Hall, 1984.

Levy, Stephen J. *Managing the Drugs in Your Life*. New York: McGraw-Hill, 1983.

Munro, Hamish N. "Nutrient Needs and Nutritional Status in Relation to Aging." *Drug Nutrient Interactions* 4 (1985): 55–74.

National Institute on Aging, U.S. Dept. of Health and Human Services "Nutrition, A Lifelong Concern." *Age Page*, 1984.

National Institute on Aging, U.S. Dept. of Health and Human Services "Don't Take It Easy—Exercise!" *Age Page*, 1982.

Prudden, Bonnie. *Bonnie Prudden's After Fifty Fitness Guide.* New York: Ballantine Books, 1987.

Roe, Daphne A. *Geriatric Nutrition.* Englewood Cliffs, New Jersey: Prentice-Hall, Inc., 1983.

Rowe, John and Robert Kahn. "Human Aging: Usual and Successful." *Science*, Vol. 237, July 1987.

Solomon, George, et al. "Psychoimmunologic and Endorphin Function in the Aged." *The Annals of the New York Academy of Science.* In press, 1987.

Soumerai, Stephen B. and Jerry Avorn. "Perceived Health, Life Satisfaction, and Activity in Urban Elderly: A Controlled Study of the Impact of Part-Time Work." *Journal of Gerontology* 38 (3) (1983).

Swartz, George, M.D. *Food Power: How Foods Can Change Your Mind, Your Personality and Your Life.* New York: McGraw-Hill, 1979.

Vitale, Joseph J., and Jose Ignacio Santos. "Nutrition and the Elderly." *Postgraduate Medicine*, Vol. 78, No. 5 (October 1985).

"Why the FDA Doesn't Crack Down." *Consumer Reports*, May 1985.

Wolford, Roy L., M.D. *Maximum Life Span.* New York: W. W. Norton, 1983.

12. WORKING ON YOUR OWN BEHALF— HELPING YOUR DOCTORS HELP YOU

American Association of Retired Persons. *Prescription Drugs.*

Brody, Elaine M., M.S.W., et al. "What Should Adult Children Do for Elderly Parents? Opinions and Preferences of Three Generations of Women." *Journal of Gerontology* 39, no. 6 (1984).

Butler, Robert N., M.D. *The Geriatric Patient.*

Miller, Roger W. "Doctors, Patients Don't Communicate." *FDA Consumer*, July–August 1983.

National Council on Patient Information and Education. "Priorities and Approaches for Improving Prescription Medicine Use by Older Americans." Draft of a report, August 1986.

National Institute on Aging, National Institutes of Health, Public Health Service, U.S. Dept. of Health and Human Services. "Help Yourself to Good Health."

Park, Constance Molino, M.D. "Medical Uncertainty and Patient Participation in Decision-Making: Truth-Telling, Autonomy, and Paternalism in the Patient-Physician Relationship." Unpublished paper, 1986.

Robb. *The Caregiver's Guide: Helping Older Relatives and Friends with Health and Safety.*

Starr. *The Social Transformation of American Medicine.*

Waitzkir, H. "Doctor-Patient Communication." *Journal of the American Medical Association* 252, no. 17 (November 2, 1984).

13. SETTING UP FOR SAFETY—DOS AND DON'TS OF MANAGING YOUR MEDICATIONS

Cooper, J. K., et al. "International Prescription Nonadherence in the Elderly." *Journal of the American Geriatrics Society* 30 (1982).

Hurd, Peter D., and Stephanie L. Butkovich. "Compliance Problems and the Older Patient: Assessing Functional Limitations." *Drug Intelligence and Clinical Pharmacy* 20, no. 3 (March 1986).

Kepler and Swisher. *The After 50 Pharmacy.*

"Medical Memory Card." *Time* Magazine, 20 May 1985.

Pepper, Claude. "Drug Use and Misuse: A Growing Concern for Older Americans." Testimony to the Joint Hearing Before the Special Committee on Aging, U.S. House of Representatives, 28 June 1983.

Robb. *The Caregiver's Guide: Helping Older Relatives and Friends with Health and Safety.*

Special Committee on Aging. U.S. Senate. "You and Your Medicines: Guidelines for Older Americans." Information paper prepared for the above committee June 1983.

Subcommittee on Health and Long-Term Care of the Select Committee on Aging, U.S. House of Representatives. "Drug

Misuse and Adverse Drug Reactions Among the Elderly.''
Briefing prepared for the above committee July 1983.

Will Rogers Institute. *Ask Your Pharmacist About Over-the-Counter Drugs*. Mamaroneck, N.Y.: 1985.

Index

About the Author

KATHRYN (KITSI) WATTERSON is the award-winning author of *Women In Prison* and *Growing into Love: Teenagers Talk Candidly About Sex in the 1980's*, both of which she wrote under the name Kathryn Watterson Burkhart. She has written extensively for magazines and newspapers, including *The New York Times*, *The Philadelphia Inquirer*, and *The Philadelphia Evening Bulletin*.